Contents

Dedication

We would like to thank our families for their support and
encouragement throughout.

Nisha Sharma and Anu Balan

Foreword

The rapid reporting section of the FRCR Part 2B examination is essentially a test of one of the most common areas of radiology – the A&E X-rays. This book will provide a very useful set of examples of cases that are likely to come up both in the 2B examination and also in a real casualty reporting pile. As the authors state in the introduction, there is a greater proportion of abnormal to normal cases in each set than occurs in the examination, but these cases illustrate the types of fractures and other cases that are used in the examination. The images are of high quality and doing these sets can be fun as well as educational.

I recommend this book as both a way of testing yourself for the examination and also as a stimulus to read more widely around some of the fractures and other cases illustrated here.

The authors are to be complimented on their selection as well as the quality of the images.

R J H Robertson MB ChB MRCP FRCR
Consultant Radiologist &
RCR Regional Education Advisor (Yorkshire)

Acknowledgements

We would like to thank Dr Chandramohan for his support and expert opinion in writing this book. We would also like to thank the following for their contributions: Dr Roderick Robertson, Dr Mike Darby, Dr Rosemary Arthur, Dr William Ramsden, Dr Marcus Nicholls, Dr Dilani Manuel, Dr Li Ng, Dr Judith Foster and Dr A Anbarasu

Finally, special thanks go to Dr Shalini Nandish for her contribution to the text and for her support.

Preface

Get Through FRCR Part 2B: Rapid Reporting of Plain Radiographs aims to help specialist registrars in radiology to pass the FRCR Part 2B exam. The book focuses on the rapid reporting and viva elements of the final phase of the radiology exit exams.

When studying for the exam, a minimum 3-month preparation period is advised. Ensure that over this period you have arranged regular practice viva sessions with as many different consultant/senior radiologists as possible. Reporting A&E films regularly prior to the exam will also help. Try to work in groups of twos and threes and practice your presentation skills with each other. Learn your differential diagnosis list for the films that you see and try to be honest when appraising each other to help you improve.

As you build up the number of vivas you are doing, you will learn techniques to deal with different and, in particular, difficult films.

In the actual exam there will be 30 films to report in 30 minutes. Time will seem to pass quickly(!), so it is important to have a system in place to deal with the films you are viewing, as there is little scope for error. During the viva, remember that your examiners will have differing approaches, but you must develop a technique that works for you. Be astute with regard to your examiner and adapt your technique should it be necessary to do so.

There are also some very good Part 2B exam courses on offer and we would recommend attending at least one of these prior to the exam, but be aware of the need to book in advance as they fill up very quickly.

This book offers seven papers, each containing 30 films, set in a rapid reporting style format. It differs in one respect from what candidates will face during the rapid reporting exam in that there are more abnormal than normal radiographs, as we wanted to give examples of a variety of pathology to convey what would be encountered in the exam. We have also included hints and tips with our answers, which we hope will be useful.

We hope that it helps and wish you the best of luck!

NS, AB

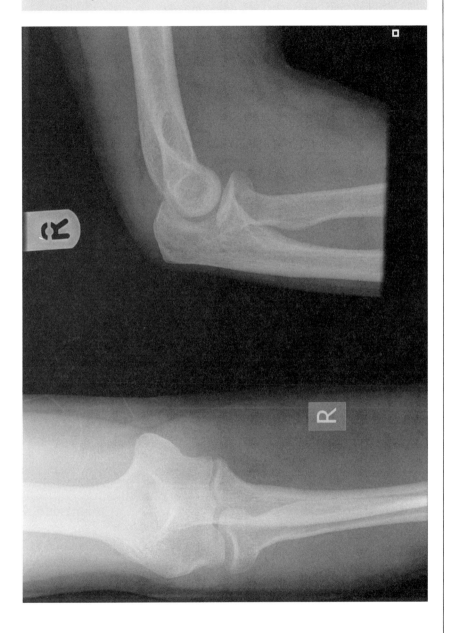

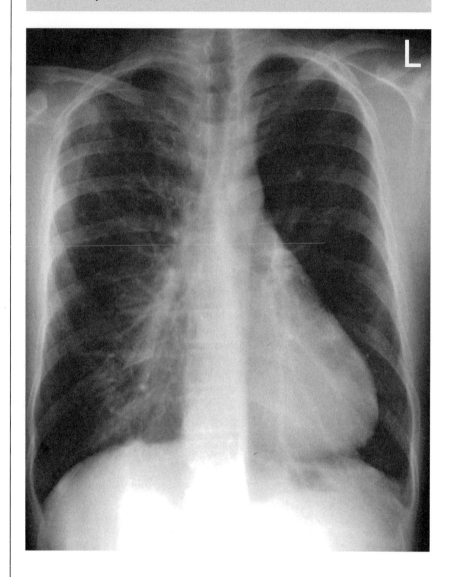

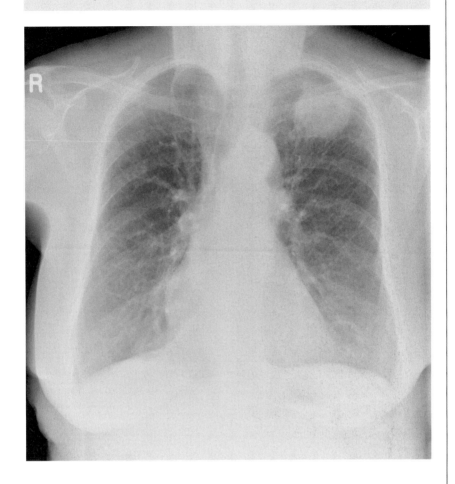

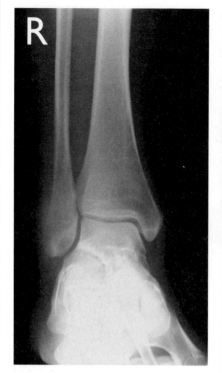
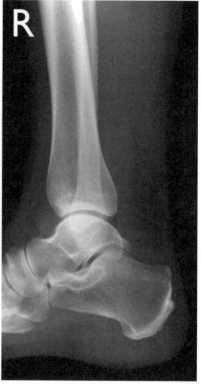

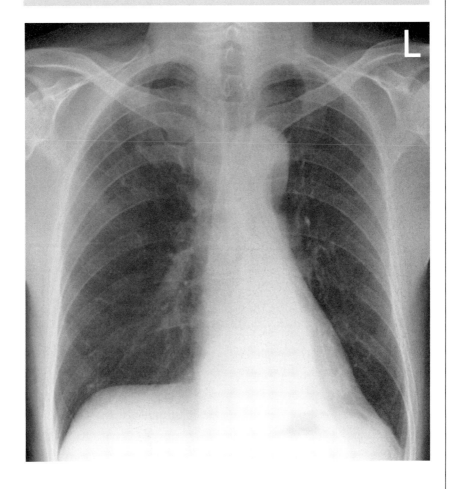

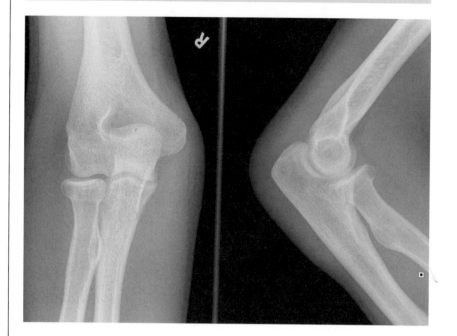

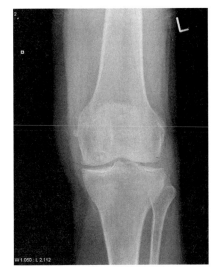
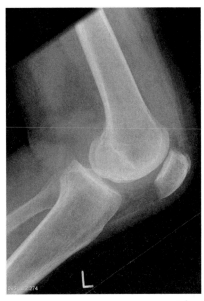

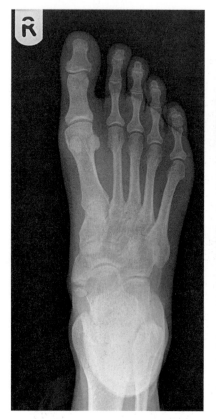
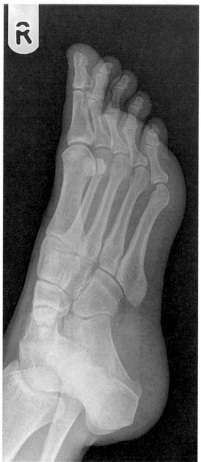

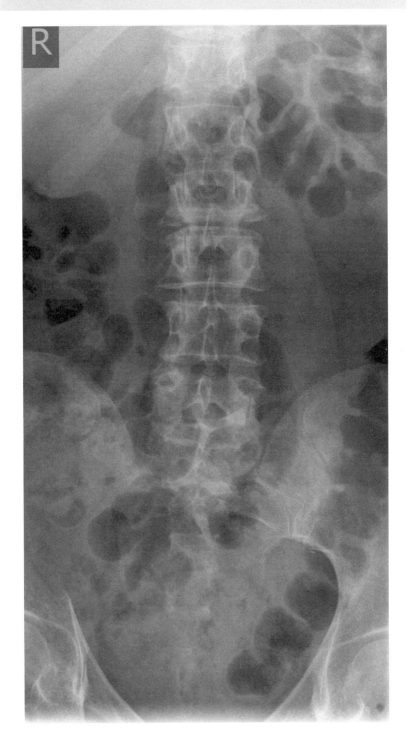

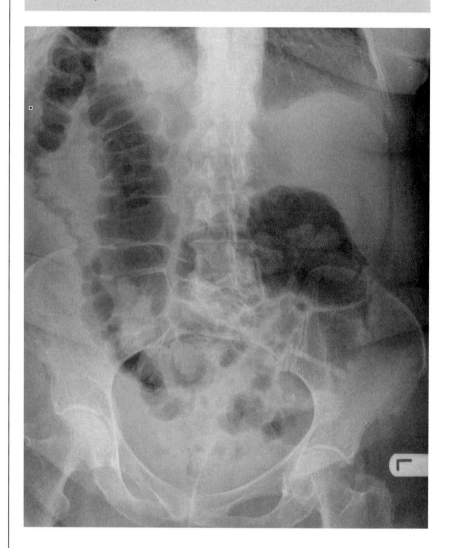

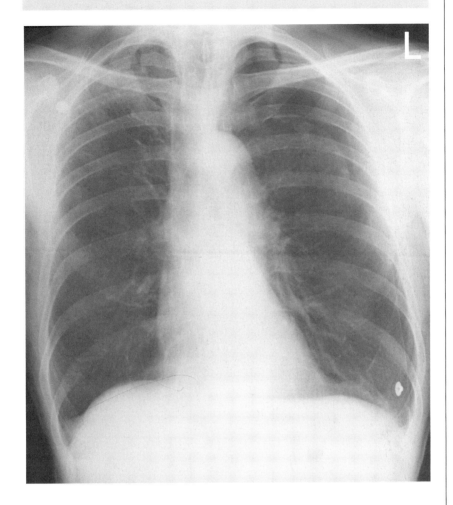

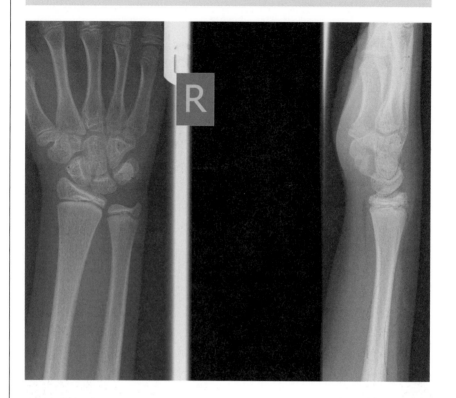

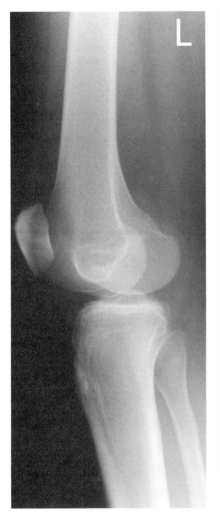 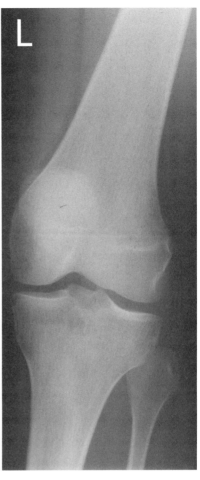

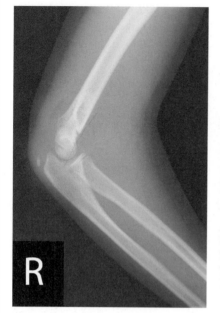

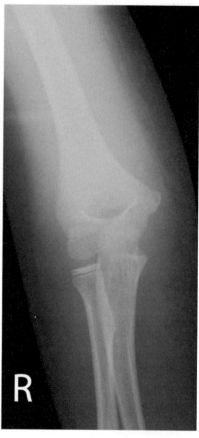

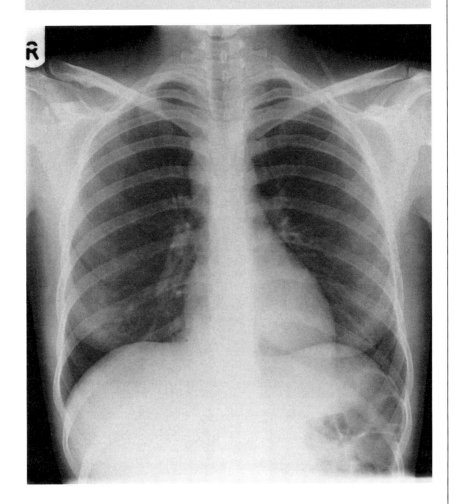

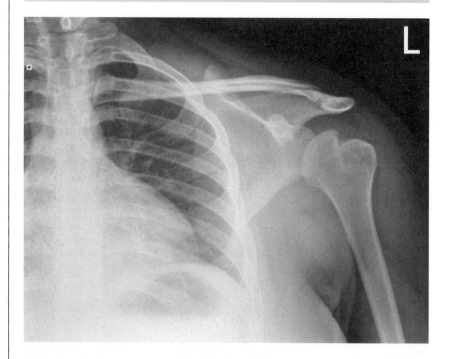

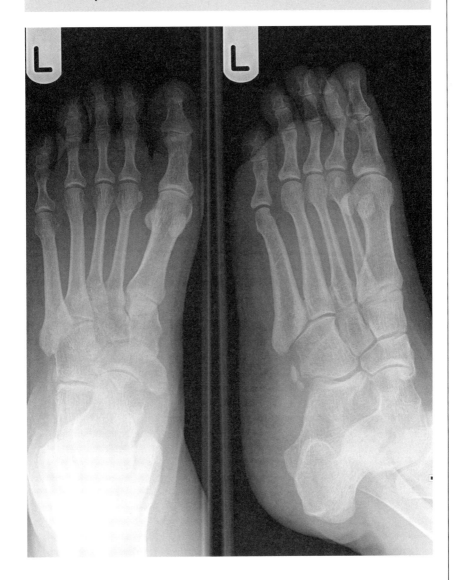

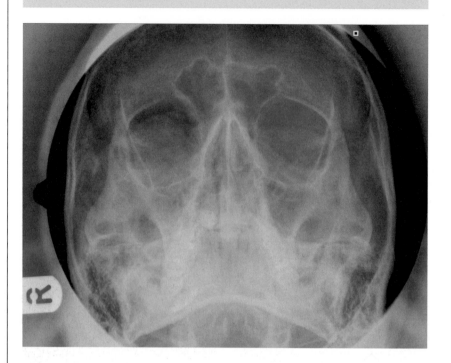

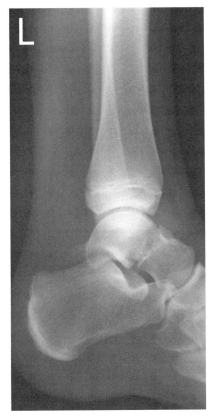
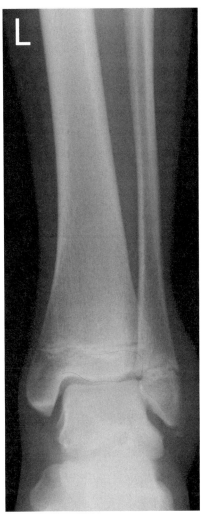

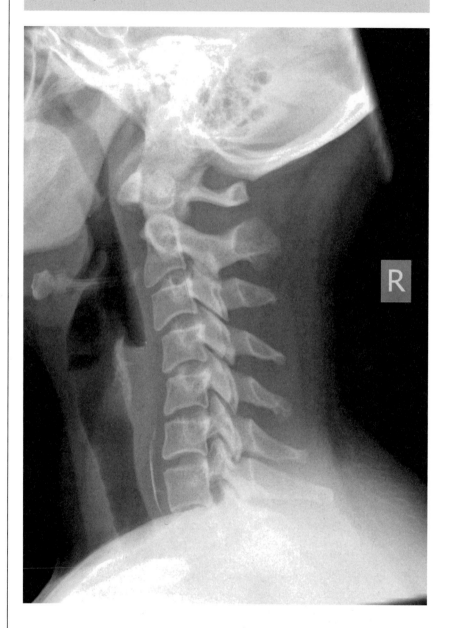

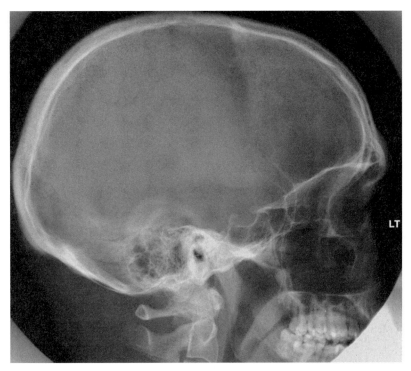

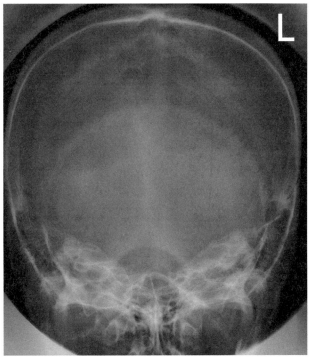

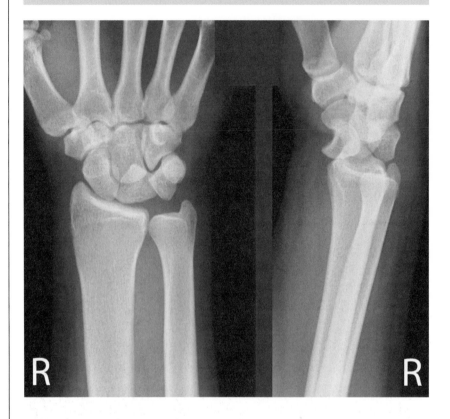

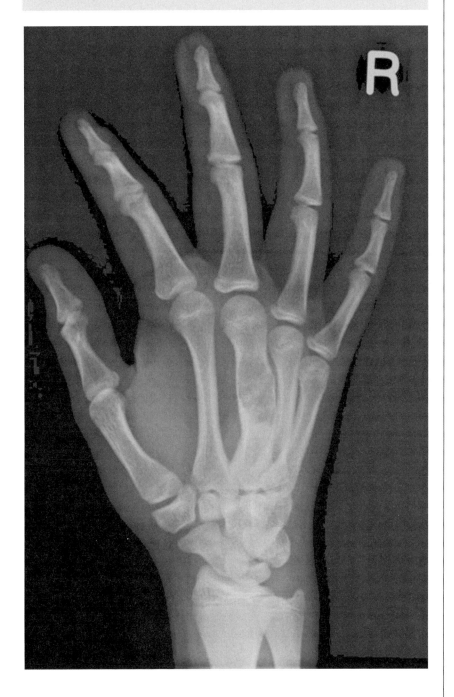

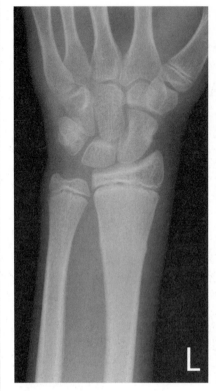

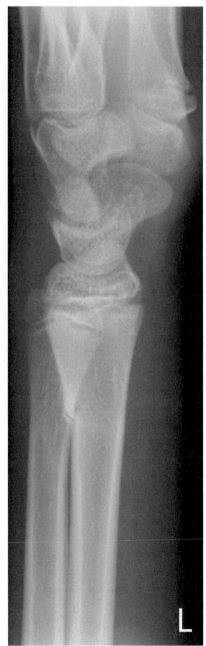

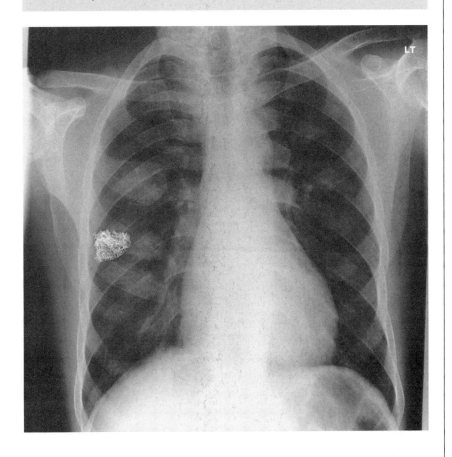

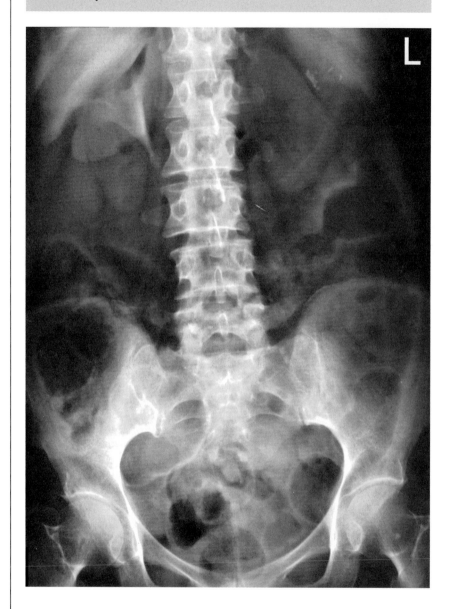

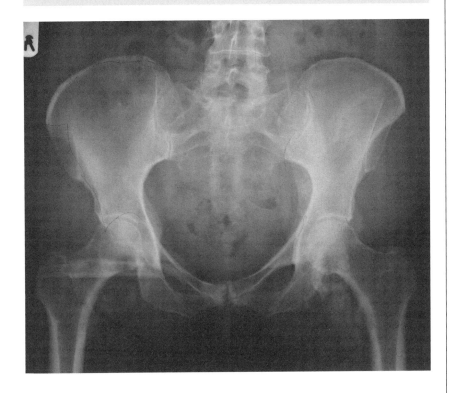

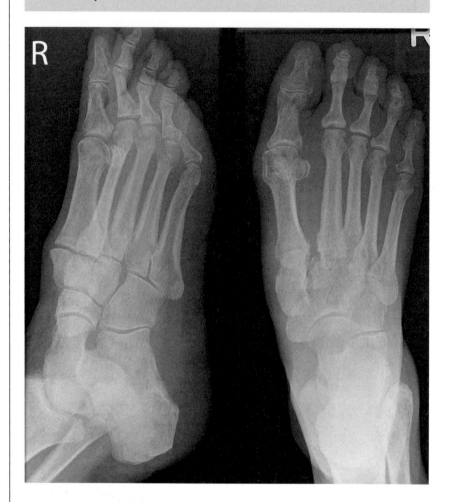

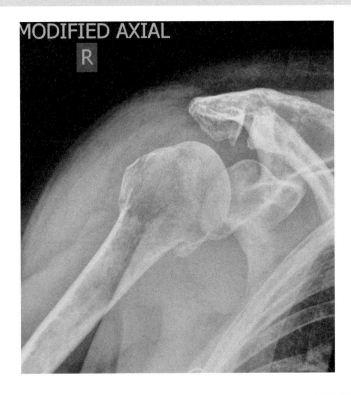

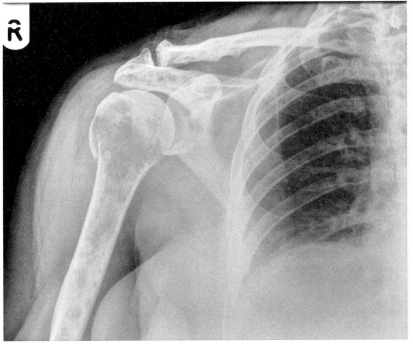

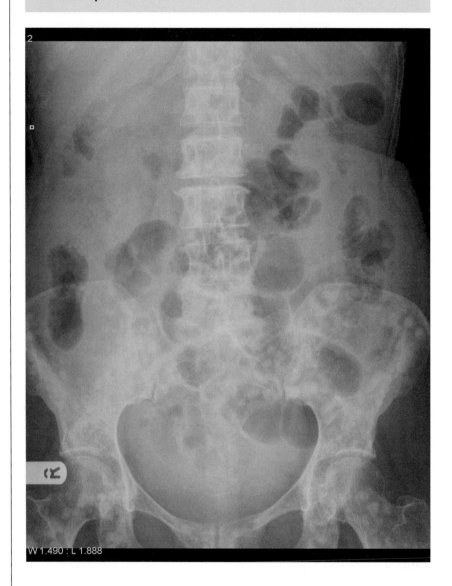

Practice Paper 1: Answers

Film 1   Right radial head fracture.

> Tip: Both the anterior (sail sign) and posterior fat pads are visible, indicating an elbow fracture and in this case a radial head fracture.

Film 2   Pectus excavatum: the sternum is depressed so that the anterior ribs are steeply and vertically orientated.

> Tip: On imaging, the right heart border is frequently obliterated because the depressed sternum replaces the aerated lung at the right heart border. The differential diagnosis is right middle lobe collapse/consolidation.

Film 3   Left upper lobe lung mass.

Film 4   Avulsion fracture of the right navicular bone.

> Tip: This occurs at the dorsal lip, at the insertion of the dorsal tibionavicular ligament.

Film 5   Left lower lobe collapse. There is a retrocardiac opacity silhouetting the descending aorta and medial diaphragm. The lateral margin is the oblique fissure.

Film 6   Normal right elbow.

Film 7   Osteochondritis dissecans of the left medial femoral condyle and an avulsion fracture of the medial collateral ligament.

> Tip: A common location of osteochondritis dissecans is the lateral aspect of the medial femoral condyle subarticular surface; it can also affect the weight-bearing surfaces of the lateral femoral condyle, tibia and patella.

Film 8 Normal right foot with os naviculare (accessory ossicle). The latter can be seen clearly in a magnified view:

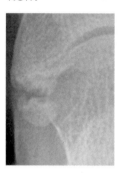

Film 9 Lytic lesion of the right iliac blade. This lesion destroying the blade is more easily demonstrated on the pelvic X-ray:

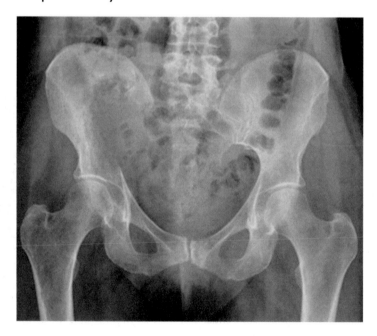

Tip: Remember to look at the rest of the film. It is hard to see what is not there! The right iliac bone is destroyed. The differential diagnosis is a primary bone lesion or metastatic deposit.

Film 10 Colitis of the ascending colon. There is evidence of thumbprinting. The differential diagnosis for thumbprinting includes ulcerative, pseudomembranous and ischaemic colitis.

Film 11 Left pneumothorax.

Film 12 Normal right wrist.

Film 13 Medial dislocation of the left patella.

Film 14 Right supracondylar fracture.

Film 15 Right paratracheal lymphadenopathy. The right paratracheal lymph nodes can be seen in the corresponding CT slice:

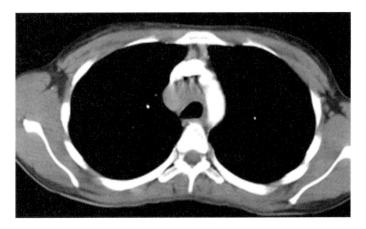

Tip: The differential diagnosis is lymphoma, sarcoidosis, TB and metastases.

Film 16 Hill–Sachs fracture of the left humeral head.

> Tip: This is a defect of the posterior lateral humeral head that occurs with anterior dislocation of the shoulder and is caused by contact between the posterior humeral head and the anterior inferior glenoid rim.

Film 17 Normal left foot with multicentric os peroneum (accessory ossicle).

Film 18 Air in right orbit: 'eyebrow' sign.

> Tip: This appearance is due to air from a sinus entering the orbit, indicating a blow-out fracture, i.e. the roof of the maxillary antrum or medial wall of the ethmoid sinus has been fractured.

Film 19 Avulsion fracture of left fibular epiphysis.

Film 20 Linear radiopaque foreign body in the oesophagus.

Film 21 Left occipital skull fracture.

Film 22 Right lunate dislocation.

> Tip: On the lateral view, the lunate is anteriorly rotated and displaced, and on the dorsovolar view, it has a triangular configuration.

Film 23 Enchondroma: third metacarpal, right hand.

> Tip: The radiographic signs are expansion of the cortex without cortical break, and no periosteal reaction or soft tissue component. Classically, this is a radiolucent lesion with internal chondroid calcification ('rings and arcs', 'popcorn' type) – 60% occur in the short tubular bones of the hands and feet.

Film 24 Torus fracture of the left radius.

Film 25 Thalassaemia major. There is abnormal bony texture with expansion of the ribs anteriorly.

Tip: Look for costal osteomas (expanded posterior aspect of ribs with thinned cortices).

Film 26 Pneumoperitoneum.

Tip: The radiographic signs are outline of the falciform ligament, a triangular collection of gas in Morrison's pouch and Rigler's sign (air outlining both sides of the bowel wall).

Film 27 Myossitis ossificans of left iliopsoas muscle. Ossification is seen projected over the left femoral head, within the left psoas muscle and also the right psoas muscle. The ossification is distinguished from malignant causes (e.g. osteosarcoma), as it is solitary and localized to skeletal muscle. It is mainly seen in young athletic adults, and can be caused by direct trauma (75%), recurrent trauma, paraplegia, burns, tetanus or intramuscular haematoma, or can arise spontaneously.

Film 28 Lisfranc fracture – dislocation of right foot.

> Tip: This is a fracture/dislocation of the tarsometatarsal joints. Look at the alignment on the normal foot radiograph; i.e. on the anterior view the medial border of the 2nd metatarsal should be in line with the medial border of the intermediate cuneiform bone, and on the oblique view the medial border of the 3rd metatarsal should align with the medial border of the lateral cuneiform:

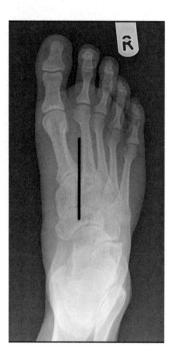 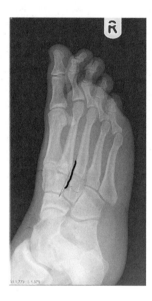

Film 29 Pathological fracture of the right humeral neck secondary to bone infiltration from multiple myeloma.

Film 30 Sclerotic metastases.

> Tip: These metastases are most commonly from prostate cancer (in adult males) and breast cancer (in adult females). They can also arise from brain, bronchial, bowel and bladder tumours and from lymphomas. They occur frequently in the vertebrae and pelvis.

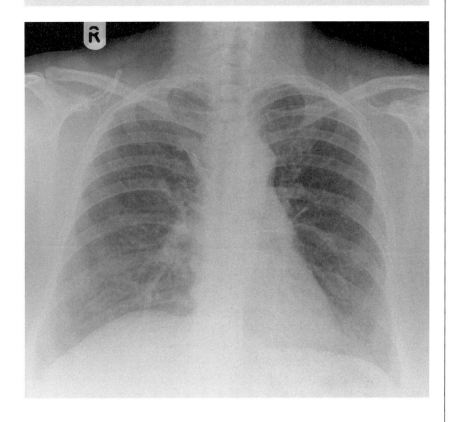

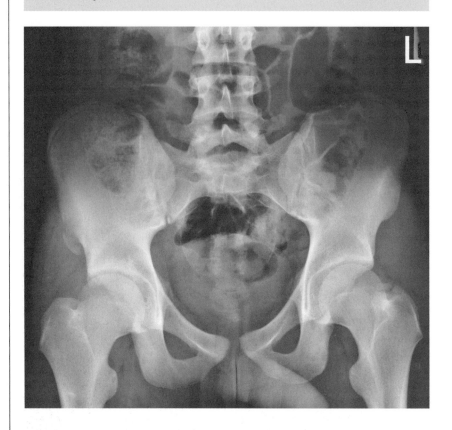

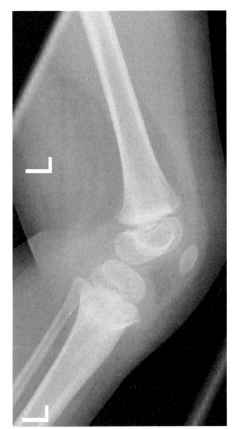 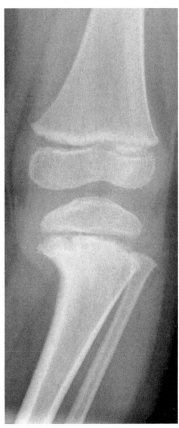

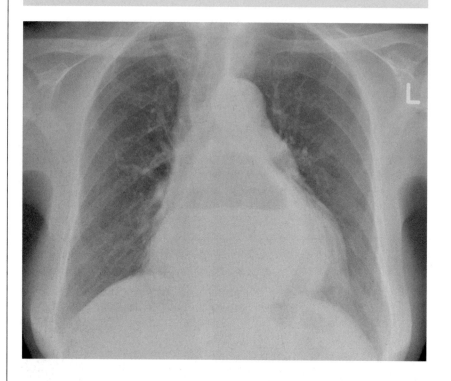

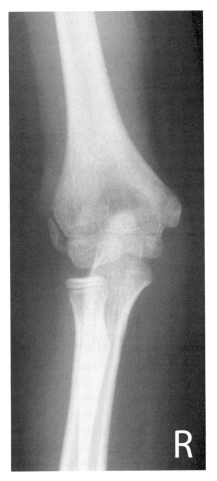
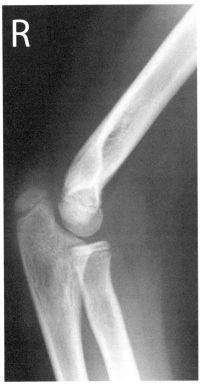

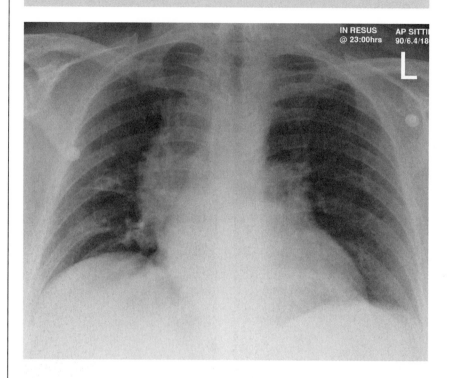

IN RESUS
@ 23:00hrs

AP SITTI
90/6.4/18

L

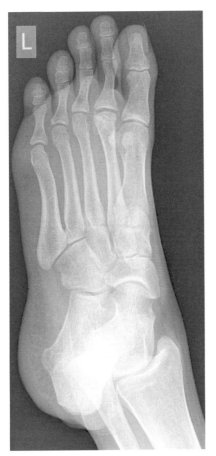
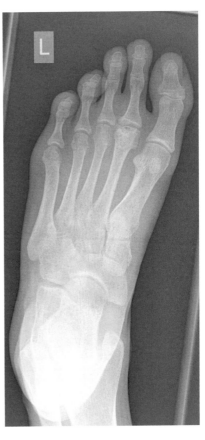

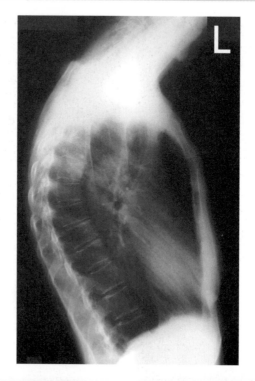

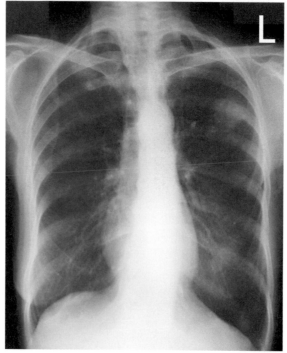

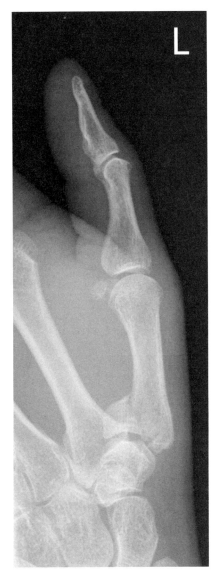
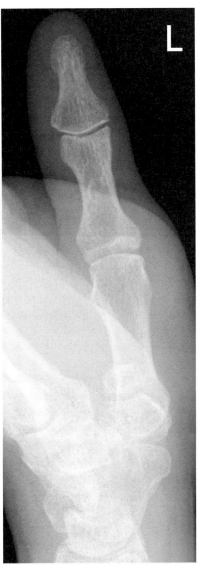

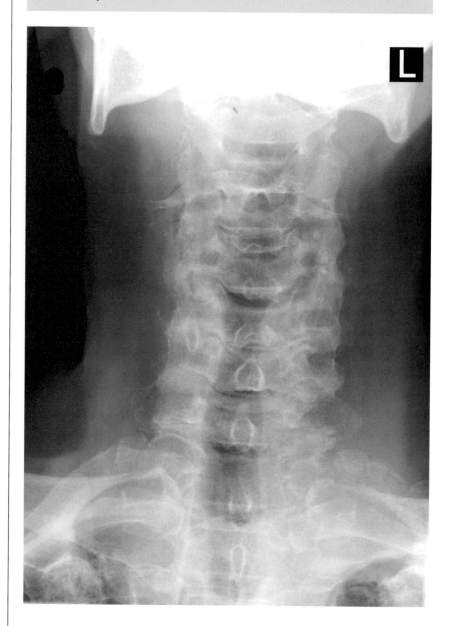

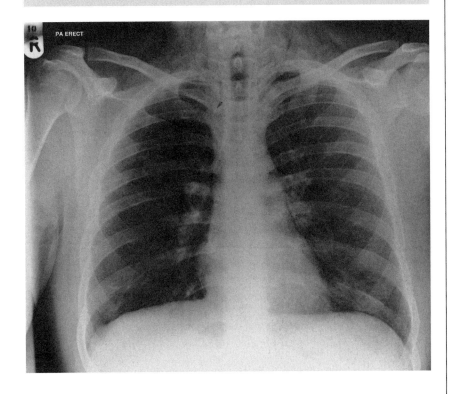

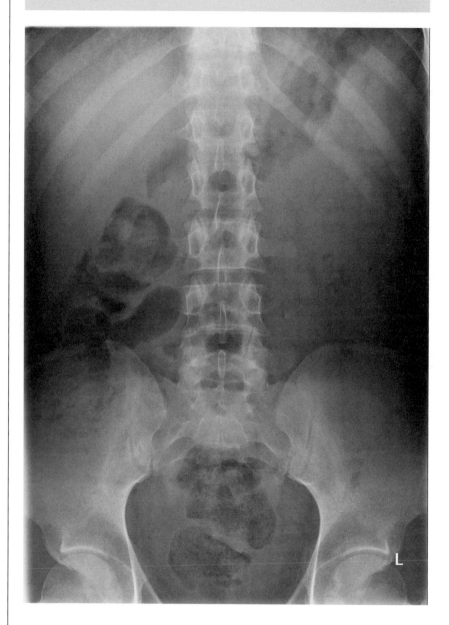

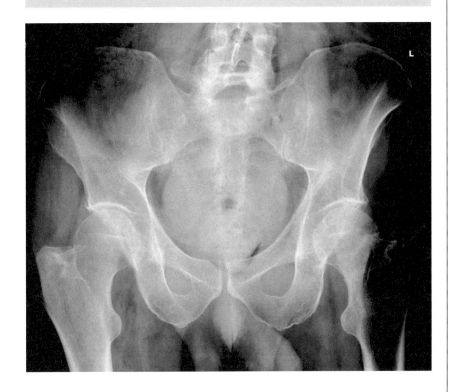

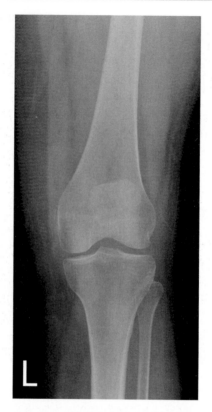

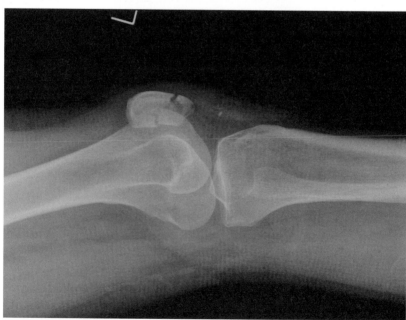

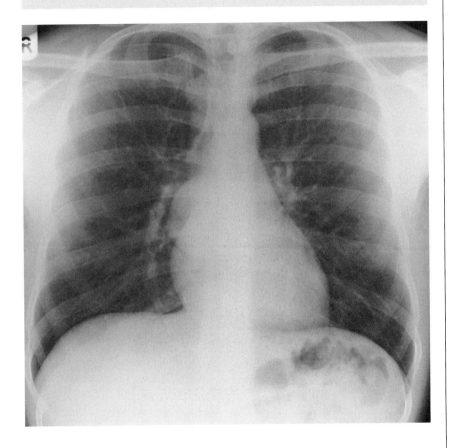

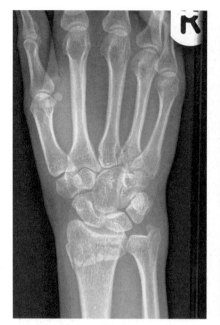
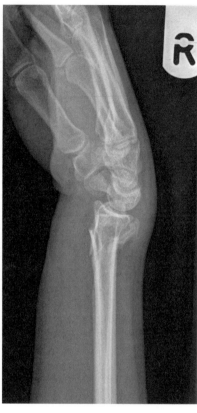

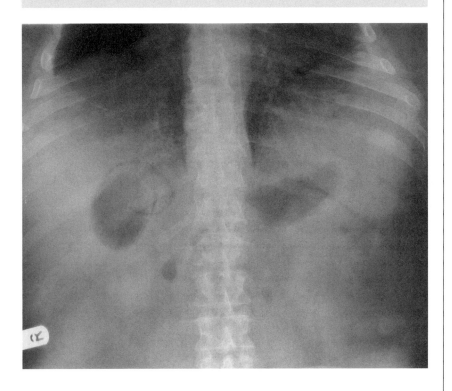

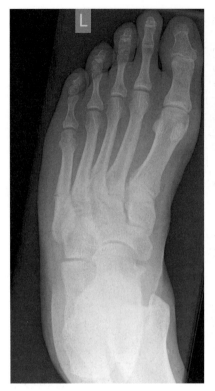
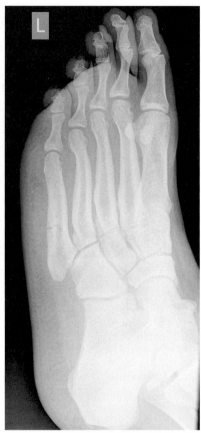

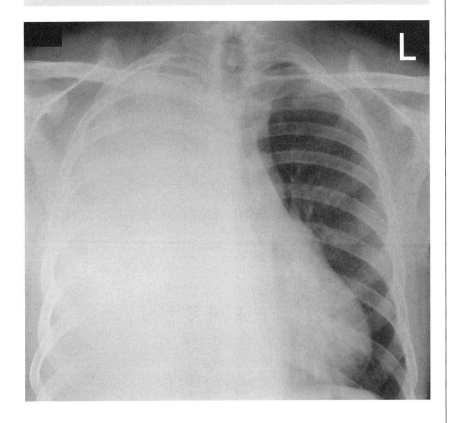

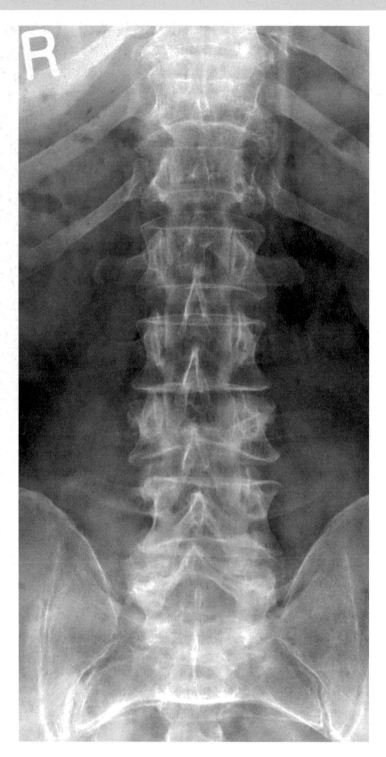

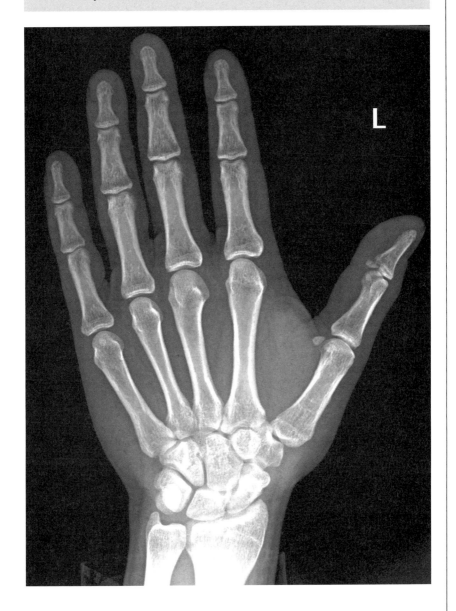

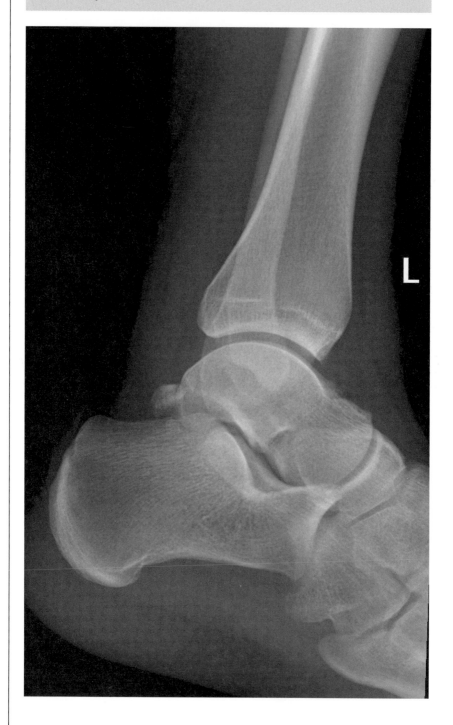

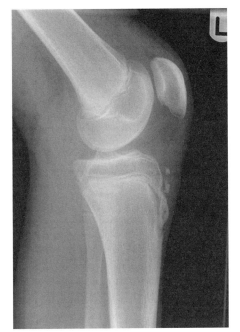 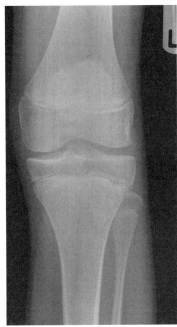

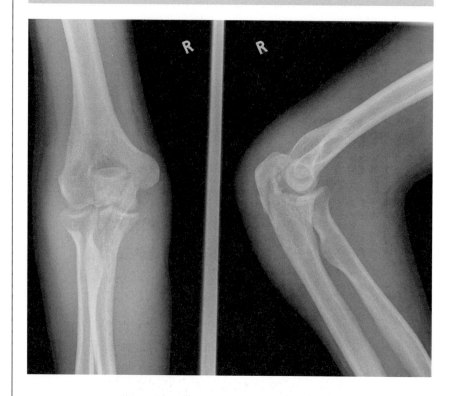

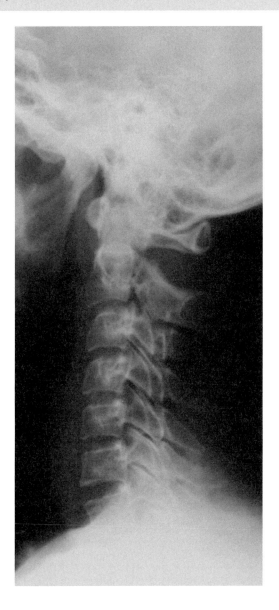

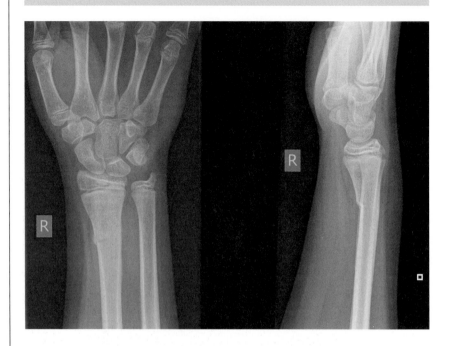

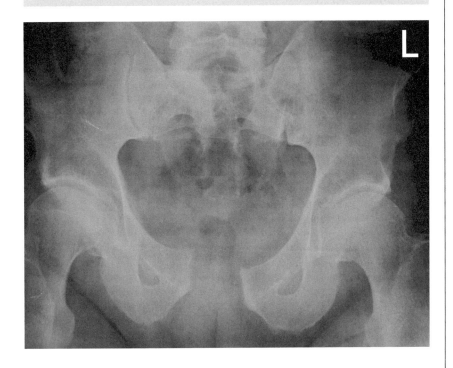

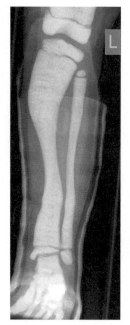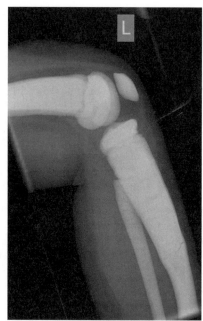

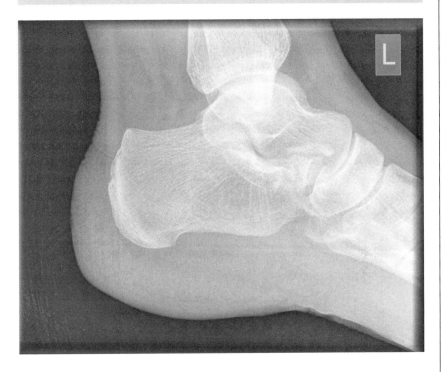

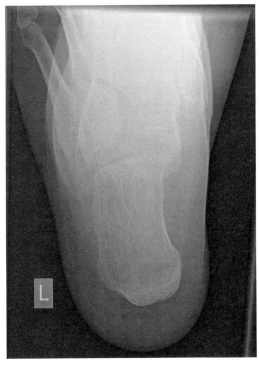

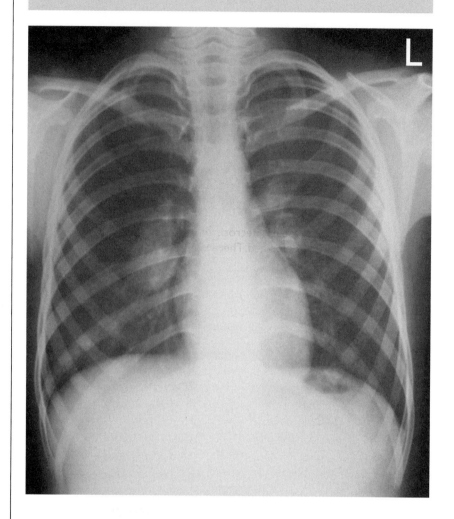

Practice Paper 2: Answers

Film 1 Normal CXR with azygos fissure.

Tip: The azygos fissure (0.5% of individuals) is composed of four layers of pleura, contains the azygos vein in its lower margin, and is invariably right-sided.

Film 2 Avulsion fracture of the right anterior inferior iliac spine.

Tip: This is the site of insertion of the rectus femoris muscle.

Film 3 Blount's disease of the left medial tibial condyle.

Tip: This is avascular necrosis of the medial tibial condyle, which is enlarged and deformed. There is beaking of the medial proximal metaphysis.

Film 4 Hiatus hernia.

Tip: Look for the air–fluid level behind the heart.

Film 5 Normal paediatric right elbow.

Tip: Make sure that you can identify and account for all five epiphyses – the mnemonic 'CRITOL' is useful in identifying the chronological order of epiphyseal fusion:
Capitellum, Radial head, Internal/medial epicondyle, Trochlea, Olecranon, Lateral epicondyle.

Film 6 Right-sided aortic arch with linear atelectasis seen in the right lower zone. The corresponding CT scan shows a right-sided aortic arch:

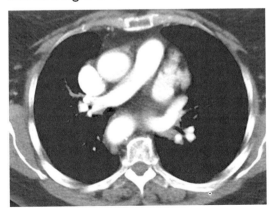

Tip: The left-sided aortic knuckle is absent. This variant occurs in 0.1% of normal adults and 6% of neonates with significant congenital heart disease.

Film 7   Freiberg's disease of the left 2nd metatarsal head.

> Tip: There is avascular necrosis of the 2nd metatarsal head. There is flattening, increased density and cystic lesions within the metatarsal head.

Film 8   Left upper lobe mass.

> Tip: There is increased density projected over the upper/mid-dorsal thoracic spine on the left lateral view. A left upper lobe mass is clearly seen on the frontal view.

Film 9   Bennett's fracture of the left thumb.

> Tip: This is an intra-articular fracture of the base of the 1st metacarpal.

Film 10 Pancoast's tumour with left first rib destruction.

> Tip: Pancoast's tumour is usually a squamous cell lung tumour. Although this case is a radiograph of the cervical spine, and therefore primarily centred on the cervical vertebrae, both apices and 1st ribs are included on this view and therefore must be included as part of the review.

Film 11 Pneumomediastinum.

> Tip: On this radiograph, the signs are subcutaneous emphysema in the neck tissues and streaky lucencies of air in the mediastinum.

Film 12 Left ureteric stone seen adjacent to the left L4 transverse process.

Film 13 Left impacted fracture of the neck of the femur.

Film 14 Fracture of left patella.

Film 15 Right bronchogenic cyst in the subcarinal region. The CT appearance of this cystic lesion is as follows:

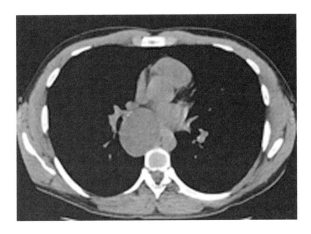

Tip: These cysts are spherical, well-defined and smooth-walled. Two-thirds are intrapulmonary and occur in the medial third of the lower lobes. Other chief differential diagnoses to consider are oesophageal duplication and neuroenteric cysts.

Film 16 Right Colles' fracture.

Film 17 Emphysematous cholecystitis.

Tip: There is air in the gallbladder wall, indicating ischaemia and infection with gas-producing organisms (diabetics are predisposed to this condition). Differential diagnoses include enteric fistula and an air-containing periduodenal abcess.

Film 18 Jones' fracture of the left 5th metatarsal.

Tip: This is positioned in the diaphysis above the tuberosity of the 5th metatarsal. Non-union is a common complication.

Film 19 Large right-sided pleural effusion with mediastinal shift.

Film 20 Burst fracture of L3 vertebral body.

Tip: On this film, the radiographic signs are loss of vertebral body height and interpedicular widening.

Film 21 Avulsion fracture of the volar plate of the distal phalanx of the left thumb.

Film 22 Normal left foot with os trigonum.

Film 23 Osgood–Schlatter disease of the left knee.

> Tip: There is fragmentation of the tibial tuberosity and associated soft tissue swelling.

Film 24 Right olecranon fracture.

Film 25 Fracture of the lamina of the C2 vertebral body.

Film 26 Greenstick fracture of the right distal radius.

Film 27 'Open book' pelvic fracture.

> Tip: This is an unstable pelvic fracture with disruption of the pelvic ring due to diastasis (widening) of the symphysis pubis and left sacro-iliac joint.

Film 28 Osteopetrosis.

> Tip: On this film, the radiographic signs are generalized sclerosis with transverse metaphyseal bands and linear lucencies from fractures due to minor trauma (brittle bones).

Film 29 Fracture of the anterior process of the left calcaneum.

Film 30 Bilateral hilar lymphadenopathy.

> Tip: Differential diagnoses for this appearance include sarcoid, lymphoma, TB, histoplasmosis and silicosis.

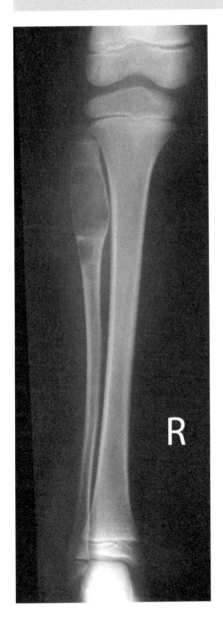

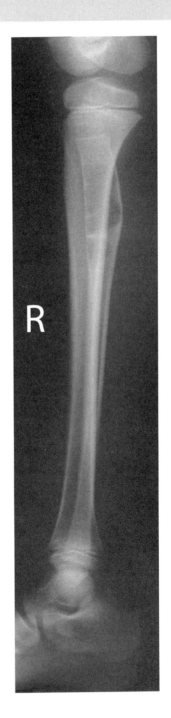

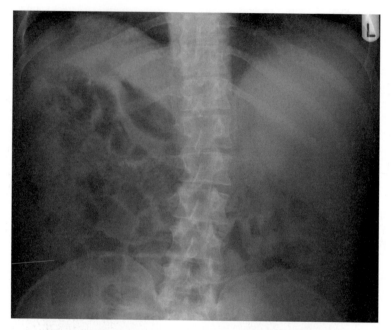

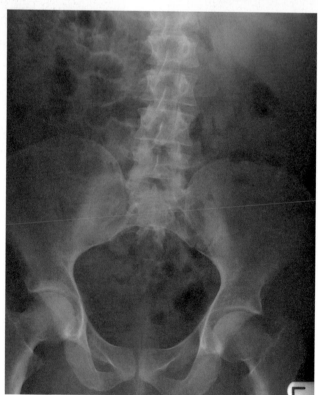

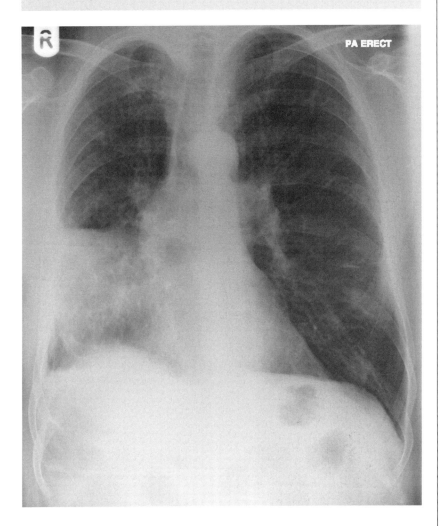

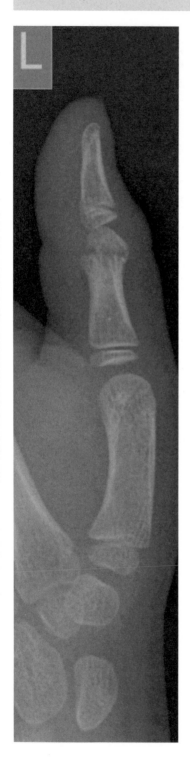
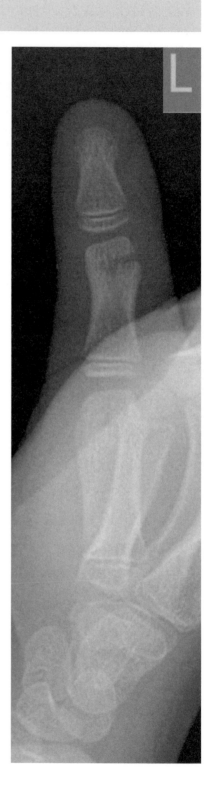

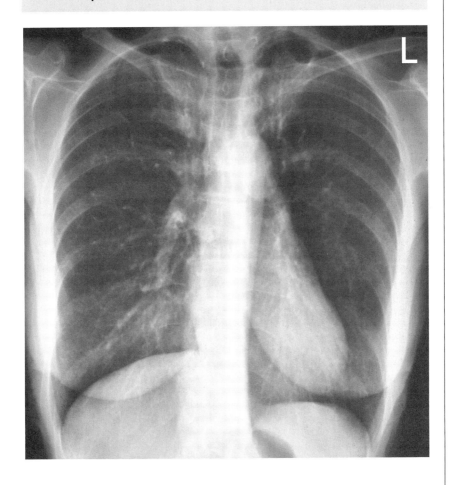

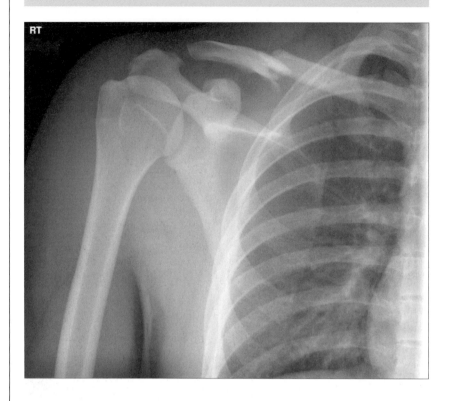

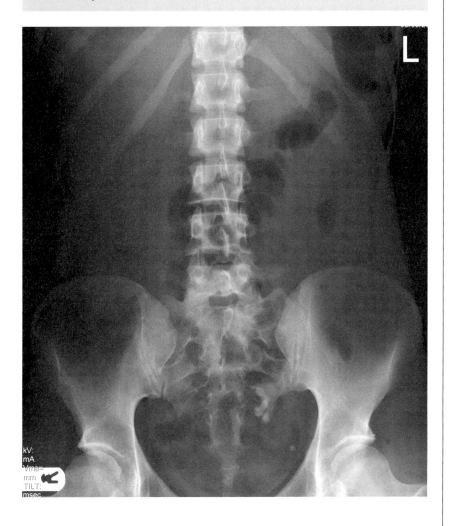

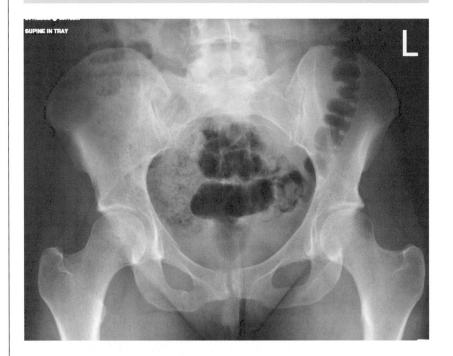

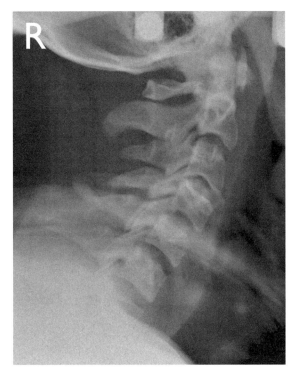

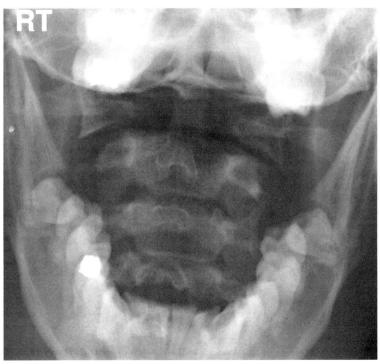

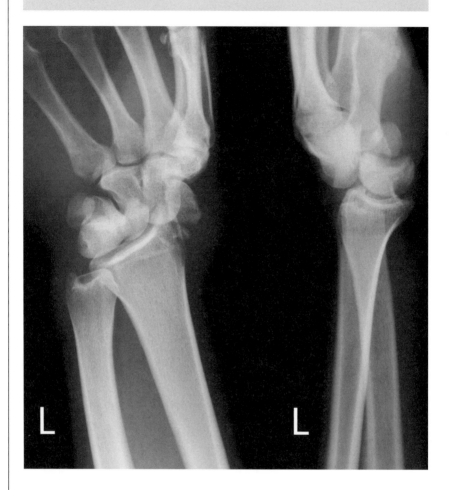

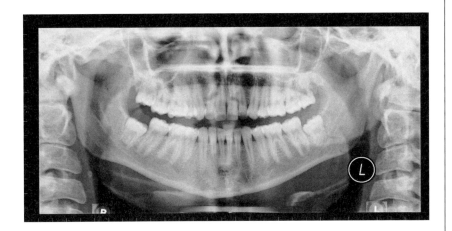

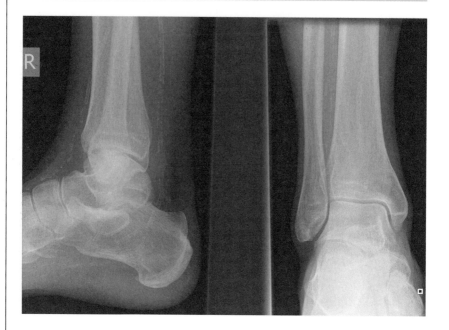

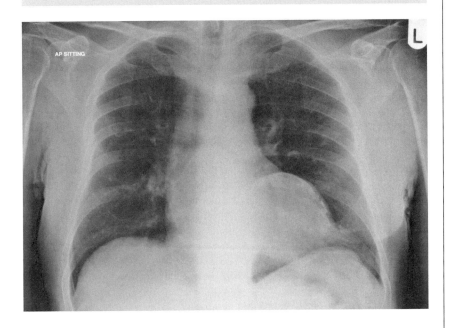

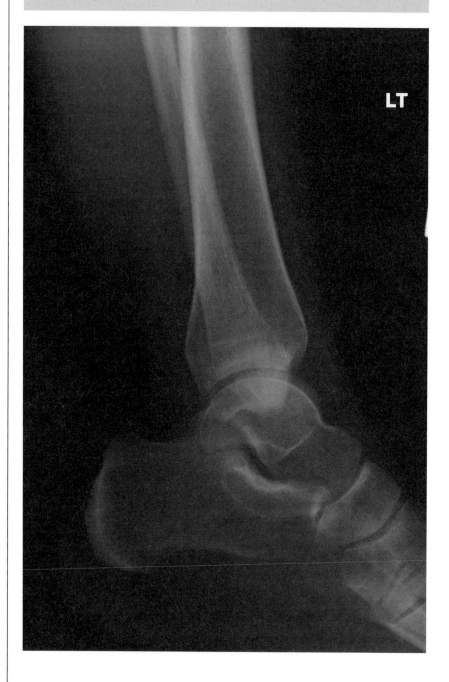

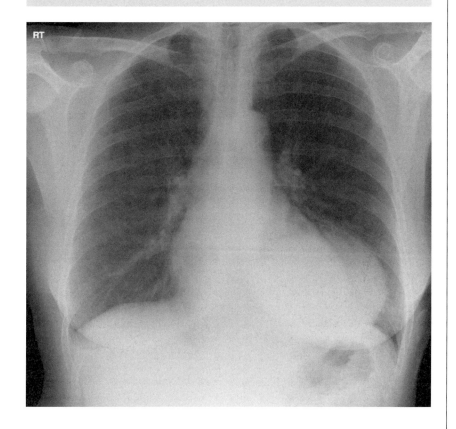

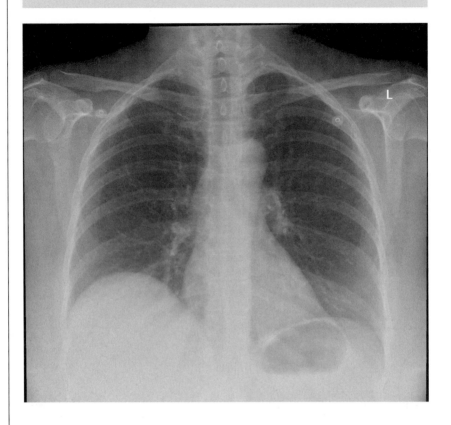

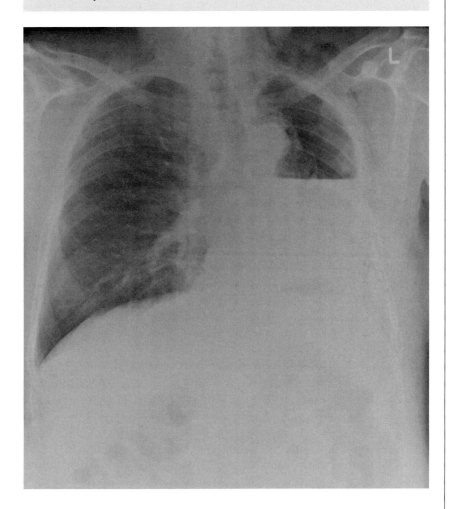

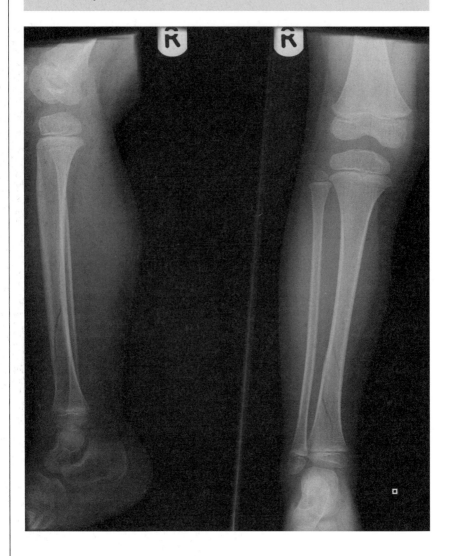

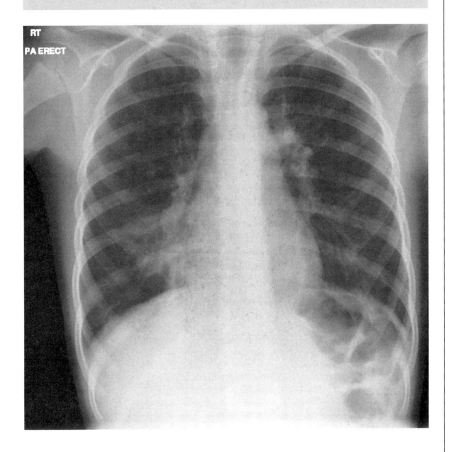

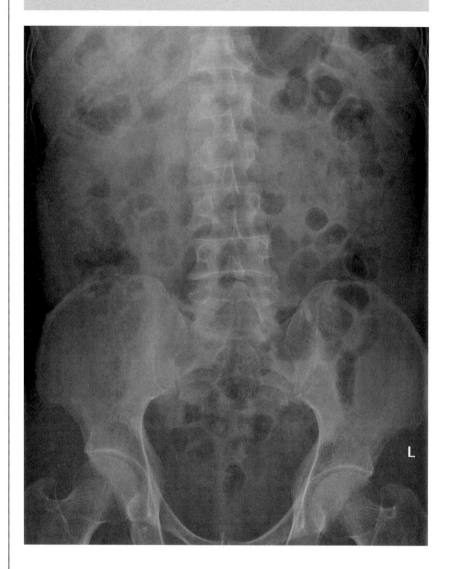

L

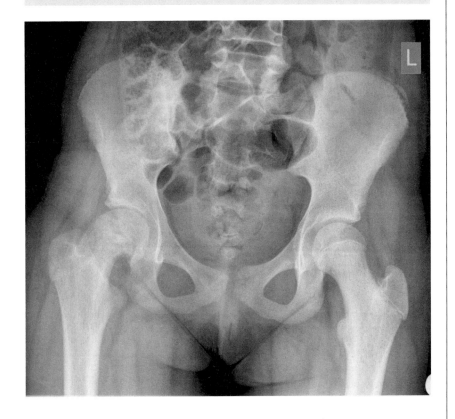

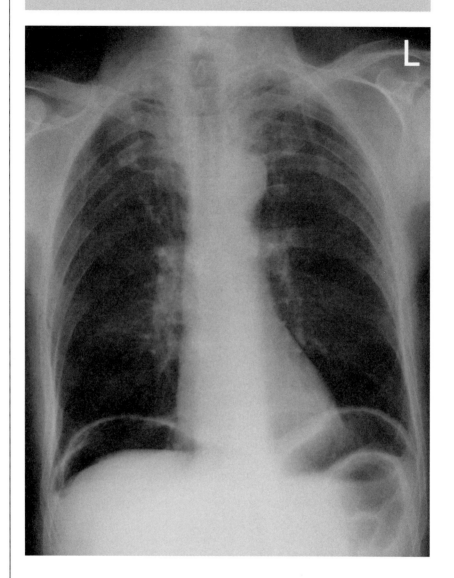

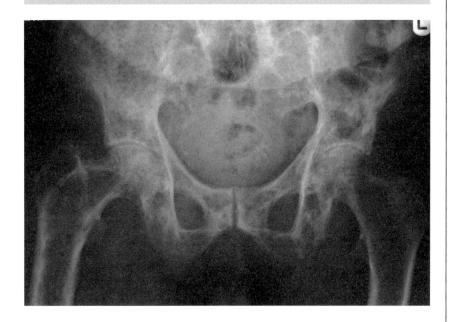

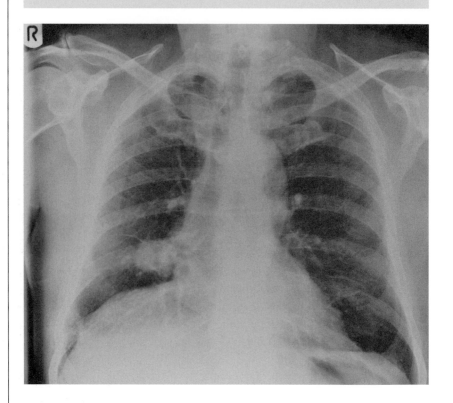

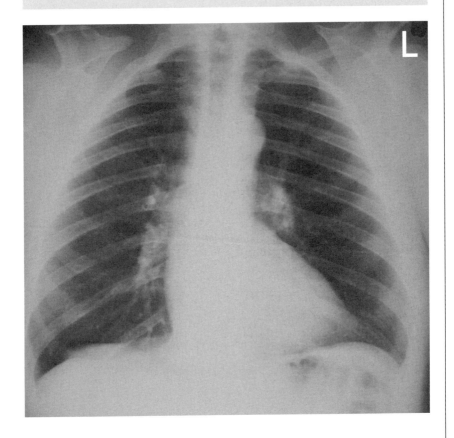

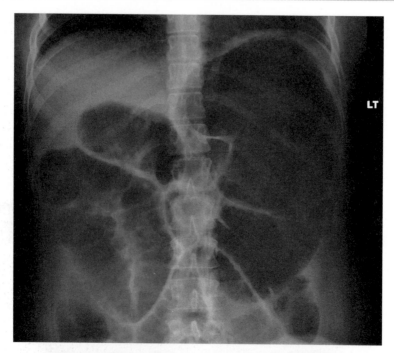

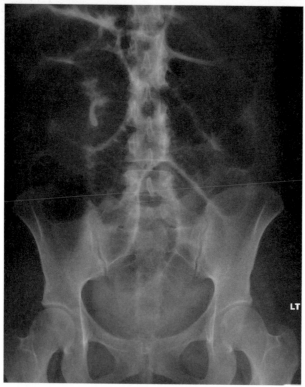

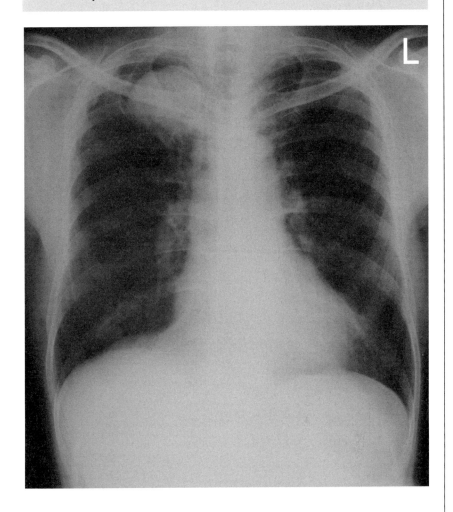

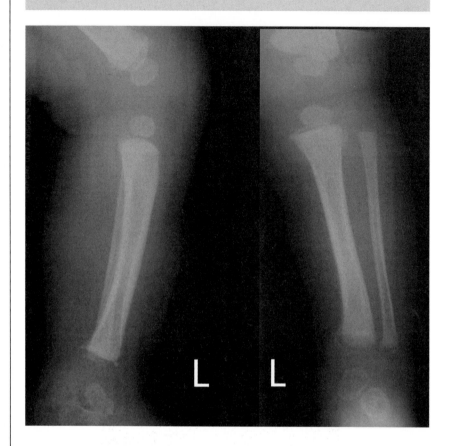

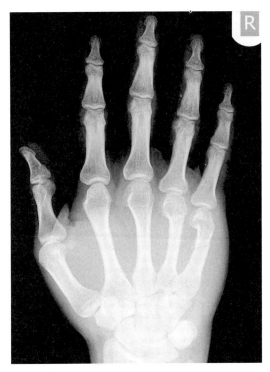

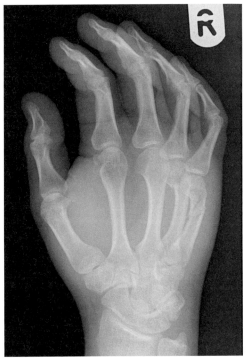

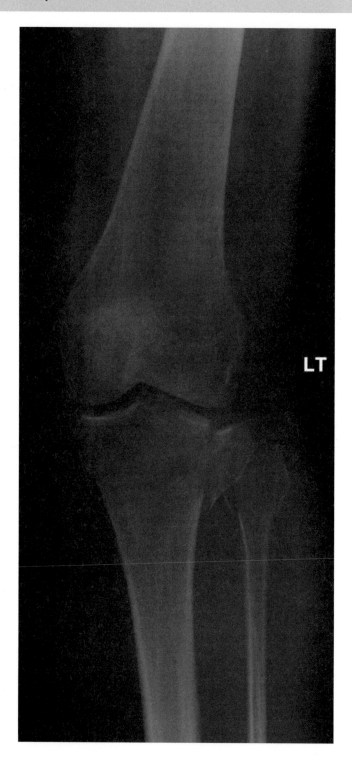

Practice Paper 3: Answers

Film 1   Aneurysmal bone cyst in the proximal metaphysis of the right fibula.

> Tip: This is a multicystic expansile lesion causing thinning of the cortex with internal septations. It is usually eccentric, but the fibula is a small bone and therefore appears central. Differential diagnoses to consider are simple bone cyst and non-ossifying fibroma.

Film 2   Situs inversus. Note the left-sided marker with outline of the liver in the left upper outer quadrant. The patient also has dextrocardia.

Film 3   Right lower lobe consolidation.

Film 4   Fracture of middle phalanx of left thumb.

Film 5   Bilateral apical fibrosis due to radiation therapy. Surgical clips can be seen at the site of thyroid surgery for thyroid carcinoma.

Film 6   Right clavicular fracture.

Film 7   Radiopaque densities seen within the left side of the pelvis suggestive of teeth, in keeping with a dermoid cyst.

> Tip: A dermoid cyst is an ovarian teratoma containing tissues derived from only ectoderm (hair, teeth, fat).

Film 8   Fractures of the right superior and inferior pubic rami.

Film 9 Jefferson's fracture.

> Tip: This is a comminuted fracture of the ring of CI (unstable). Both articular pillars of CI are offset laterally versus those of C2 on an open-mouth view.

Film 10 Left perilunate dislocation.

> Tip: This is two to three times more common than lunate dislocation.

Film 11 Left mandibular fracture.

Film 12 Normal right ankle with vascular calcification.

Film 13 Calcified left ventricular aneurysm.

Film 14 Left base of 5th metatarsal fracture.

> Tip: This was an ankle X-ray, but remember to look at the rest of the bones.

Film 15 Left posterior mediastinal mass. The corresponding CT scan shows a large cystic lesion in the posterior mediastinum:

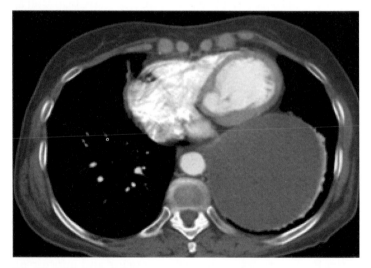

> Tip: The differential diagnoses are neurogenic tumour, vascular mass, foregut cyst and extramedullary haematopoeisis. This case was a foregut cyst.

Film 16 Normal chest.

Film 17 Left hydropneumothorax with surgical emphysema.

Film 18 Spiral fracture of right tibia.

Film 19 Right middle lobe consolidation.

Film 20 Normal abdomen.

Film 21 Slipped right capital femoral epiphysis.

> Tip: There is posteromedial displacement of the femoral head. The line of Klein (a line drawn along the superior edge of the femoral neck) fails to intersect the femoral head. The epiphysis appears smaller due to posterior slippage. Males are affected more than females.

Film 22 Pneumoperitoneum.

Film 23 Paget's disease of the pelvis and right proximal femur. There is a pathological right intertrochanteric fracture.

Film 24 Right lower lobe mass.

Film 25 Cleidocranial dysostosis.

> Tip: The right clavicle is absent and there is hypoplasia of the left clavicle. The thorax is narrowed and bell-shaped. This can also be associated with supernumerary ribs.

Film 26 Caecal volvulus with small bowel obstruction.

> Tip: The 'kidney-shaped' distended caecum lies in the left upper outer quadrant. Males are more commonly affected than females. It is associated with malrotation and a long mesentery.

Film 27 Right mycetoma.

> Tip: There is a fungus ball lying within a pre-existing cavity. The causative organism is usually Aspergillus. Often, the cavity is due to prior TB or sarcoidosis. The 'air crescent' sign is typical of mycetoma.

Film 28 'Bucket handle' fractures of the distal left femur, proximal and distal tibia, and distal fibula.

> Tip: These are very specific for non-accidental injury. They involve the metaphysis. They are most common in the lower femur, upper and lower tibia, and upper humerus.

Film 29 Fracture of the shaft of the 5th right metacarpal.

Film 30 Fracture of the left lateral tibial plateau and fibular neck.

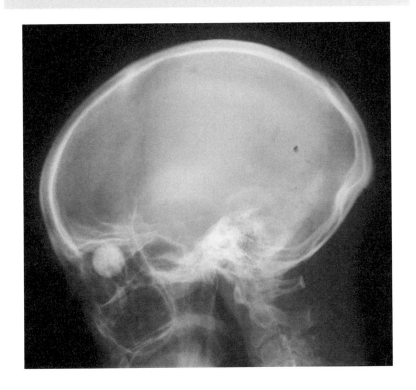

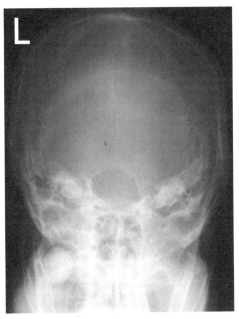

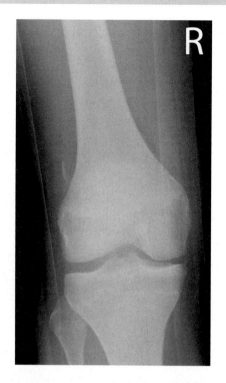

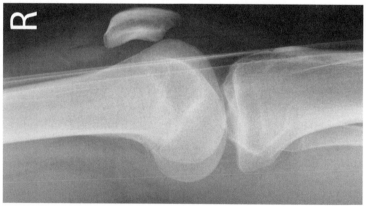

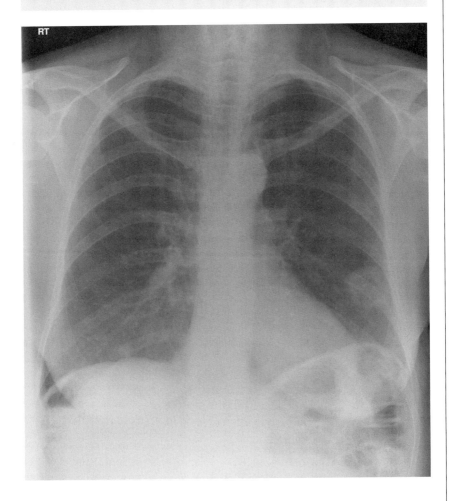

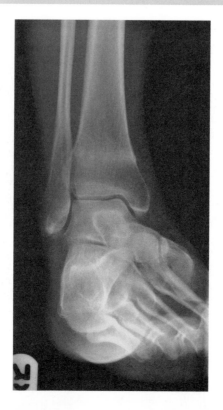

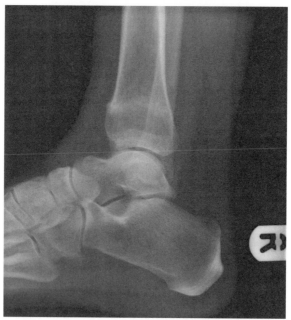

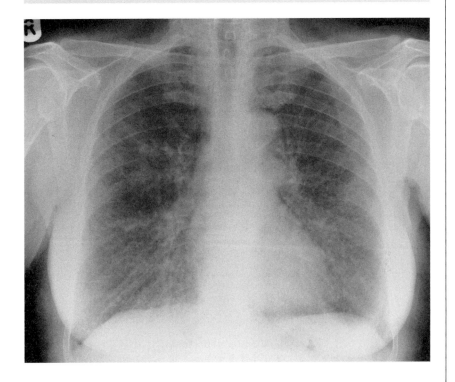

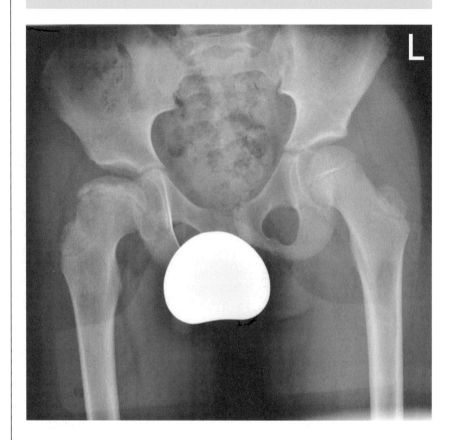

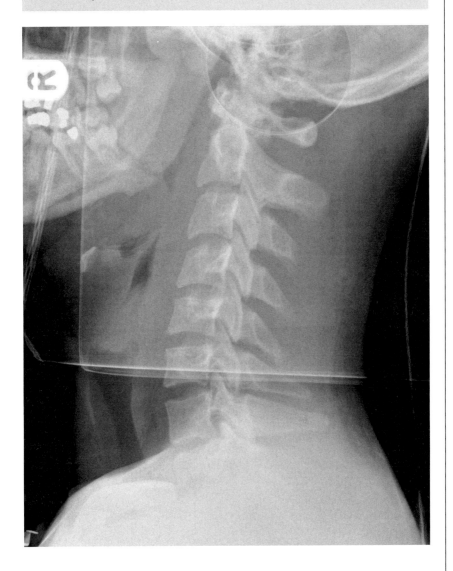

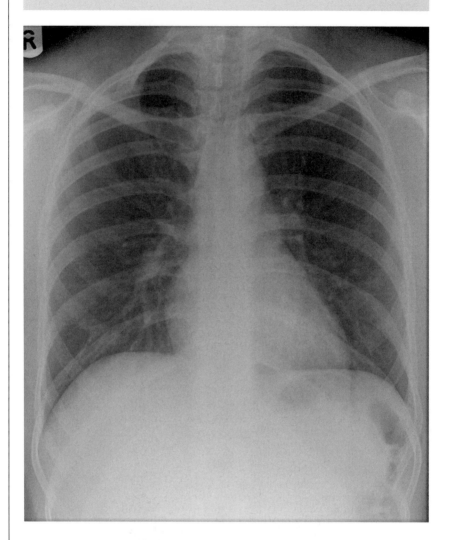

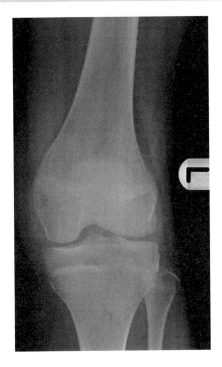

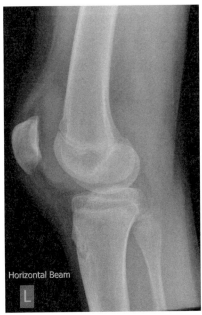

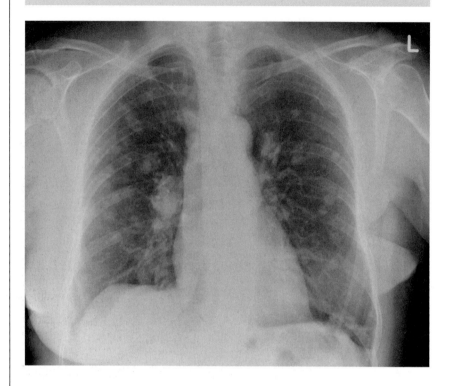

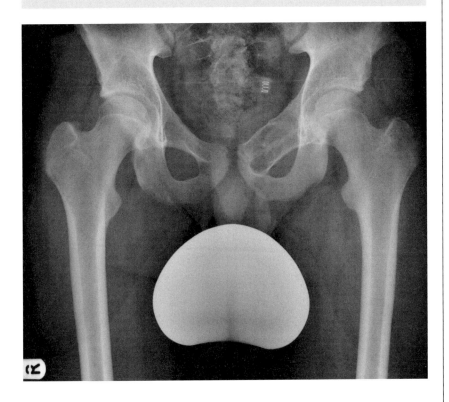

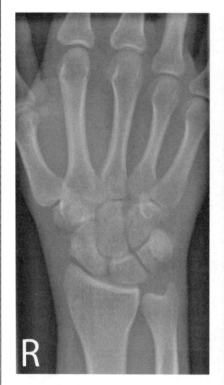
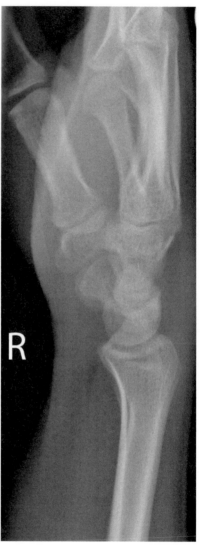

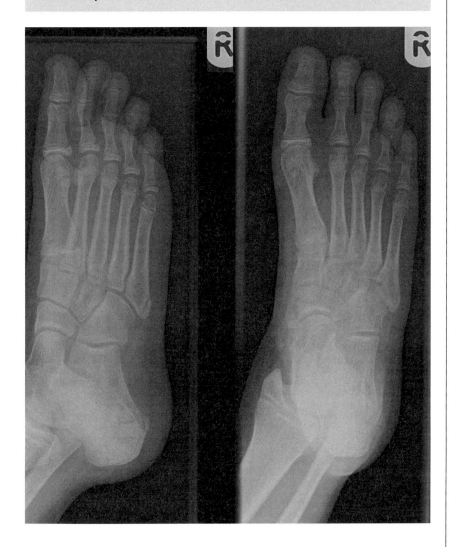

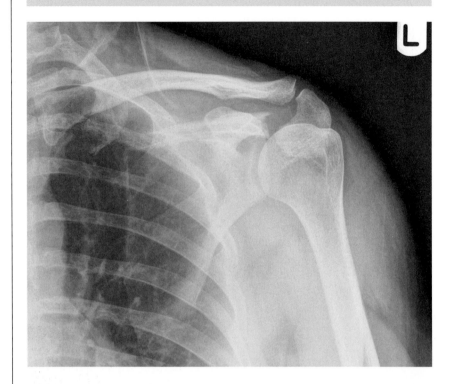

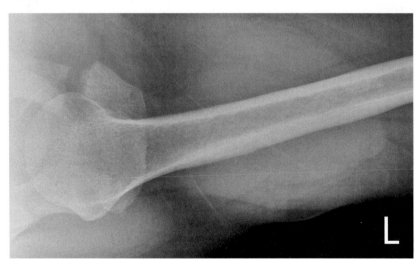

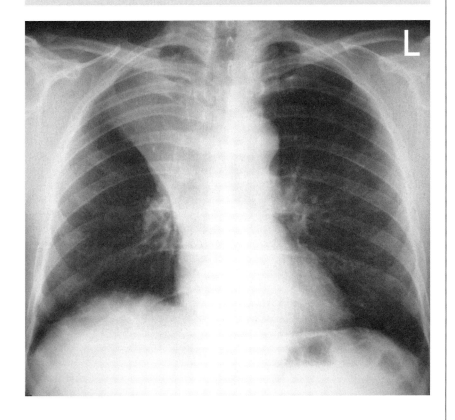

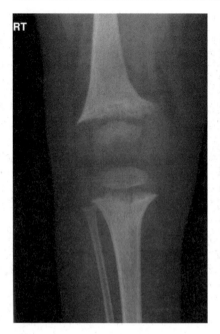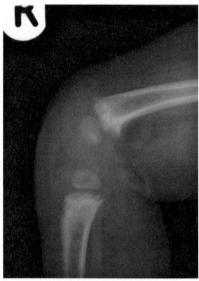

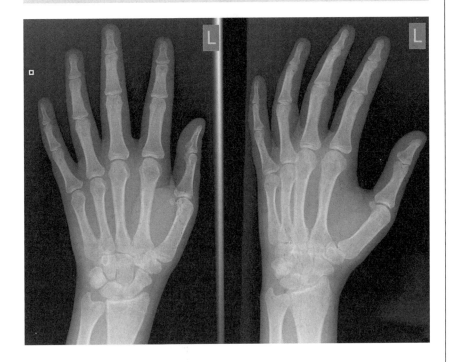

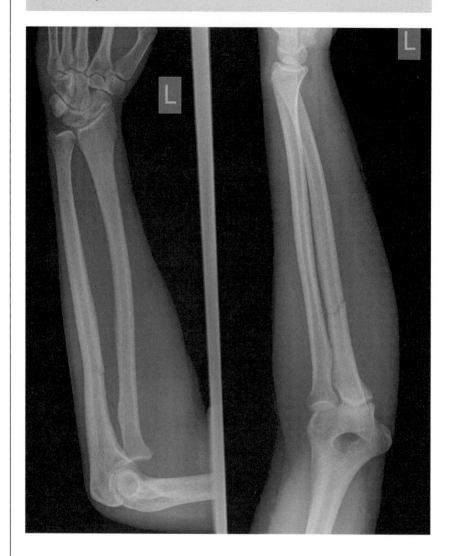

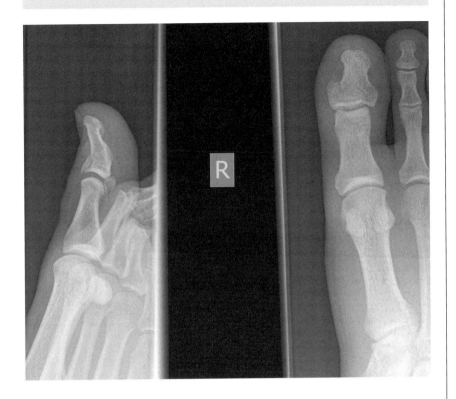

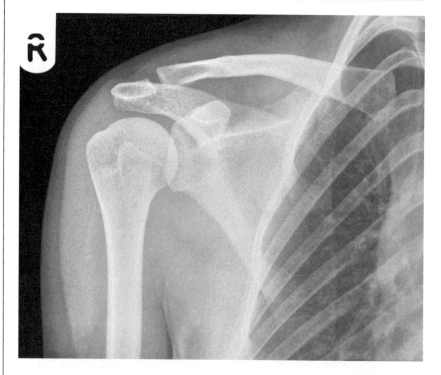

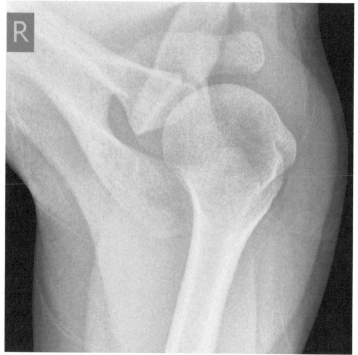

124

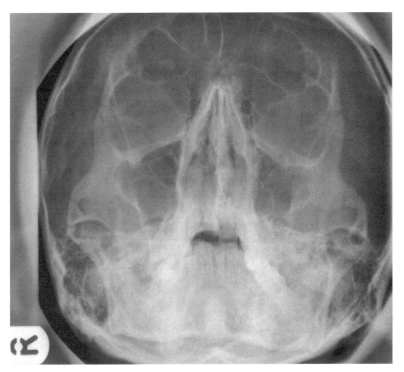

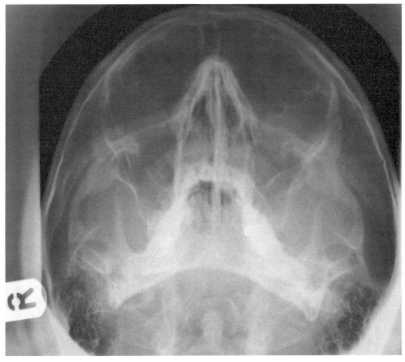

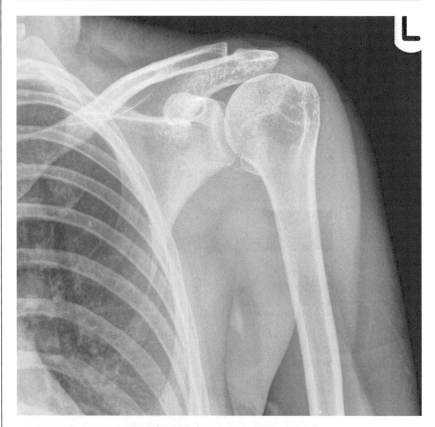

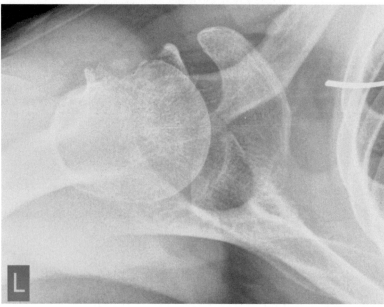

126

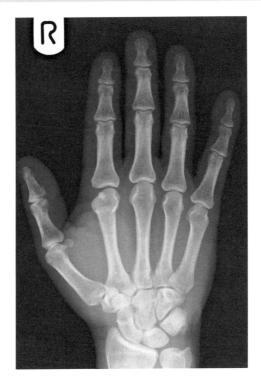

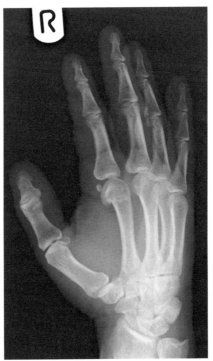

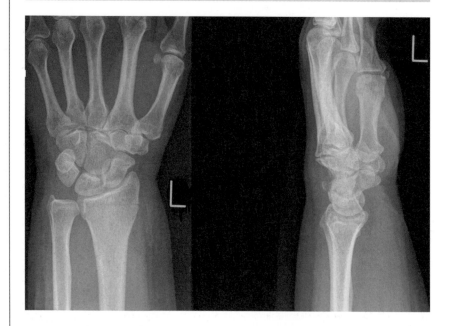

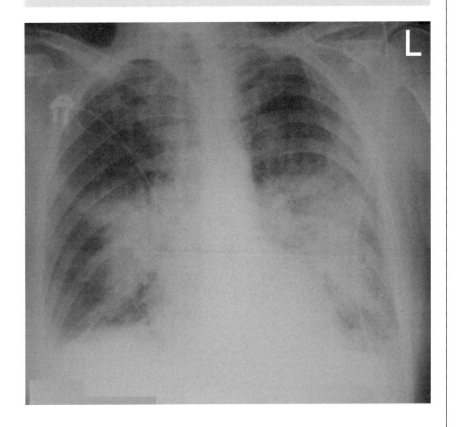

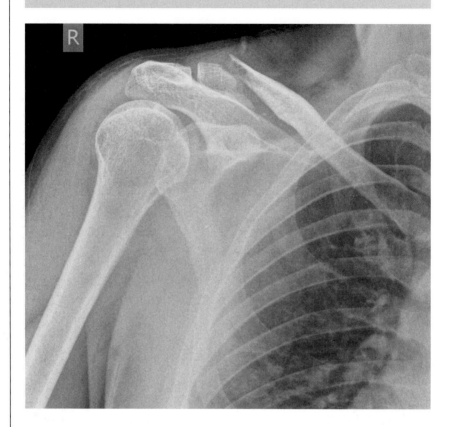

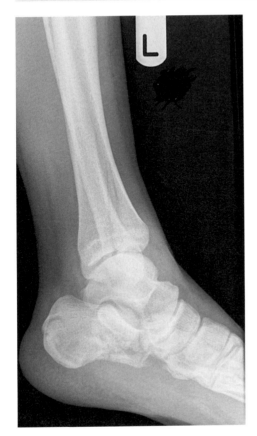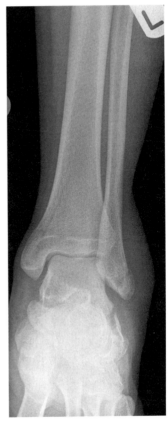

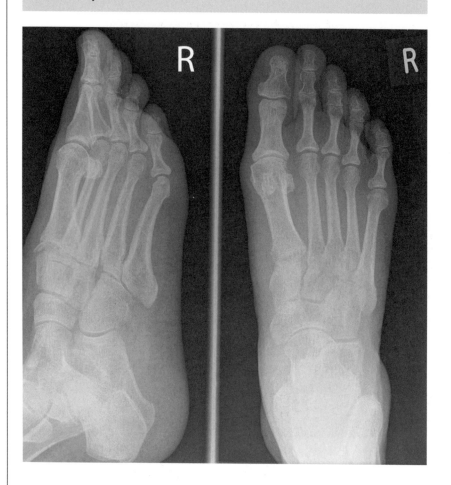

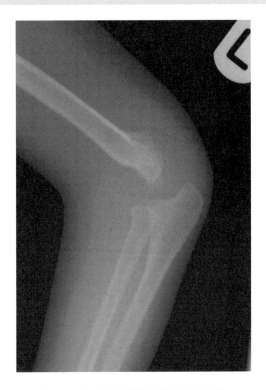

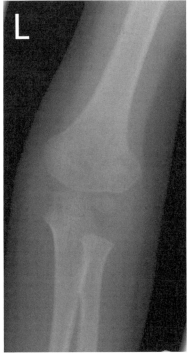

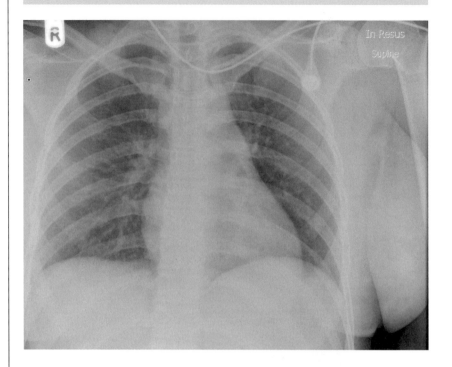

Practice Paper 4: Answers

Film 1   Normal skull. The round radiopaque foreign body in the left orbital cavity is a glass eye.

Film 2   Osteochondral fracture with lipohaemarthrosis of the right knee.

Film 3   Wegener's granulomatosis. There are several nodules in the mid- and lower zones, with a cavitating lesion in the left lower lobe. The corresponding CT scan shows several cavitating lesions:

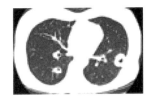

Tip: Lung nodules tend to be bronchocentric, or subpleural and peripheral. 50% of lung nodules and masses cavitate.
Cavities are often thick-walled. When multiple, they are usually less than 10 in number.

Film 4   Right tibial stress fracture with sclerosis.

Tip: Tibial shaft stress fractures tend to occur in runners, ballet dancers and other athletes (19–63%). Cancellous bone sclerosis is seen in the inferior metadiaphysis.

Film 5   Lymphangitis carcinomatosis.

Tip: Reticulonodular opacities, coarse bronchovascular markings, septal lines and Kerley B lines. Differential diagnoses to consider are pulmonary oedema, idiopathic pulmonary fibrosis, lymphoma and sarcoidosis.

Film 6 Right Perthes' disease.

> Tip: There is flattening, sclerosis and fragmentation of the right femoral capital epiphysis.

Film 7 Bilateral rami fractures of the mandible on a lateral C-spine view. The fractures are more evident on a mandibular view:

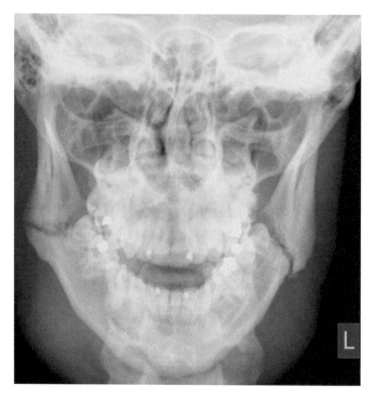

> Tip: The lateral C-spine is normal. Remember to look at the whole film.

Film 8 Normal chest with cervical ribs.

Film 9 Avulsion fracture of the inferior pole of the left patella with large joint effusion.

Film 10 Lung metastases. Left mastectomy with surgical clips in left axilla.

Film 11 Aneurysmal bone cyst of the left superior pubic ramus.

Film 12 Right scaphoid fracture.

Film 13 Normal right foot.

> Tip: The epiphysis of the 5th metatarsal is normal. The long axis of the unfused apophysis runs parallel to the metatarsal.

Film 14 Fracture of the acromion of the left scapula.

Film 15 Right upper lobe collapse.

Film 16 Rickets of right knee.

> Tip: There is splaying, fraying and widening of the metaphyses. There is widening of the epiphyses.

Film 17 Normal left hand.

Film 18 Left Monteggia fracture.

> Tip: This is a fracture of the shaft of the ulna and dislocation of the radial head, which is identified by an abnormal radiocapitellar line.

Film 19 Intra-articular fracture of the base of the distal phalanx of the right great toe.

Film 20 Normal right shoulder.

Film 21 Left tripod fracture.

> Tip: There is widening of the zygomatico-frontal suture, fracture of the zygomatic arch and fracture through the body of the zygoma.

Film 22 Fracture of the lesser tuberosity of the left humerus.

Film 23 Fracture of the neck of the 2nd right metacarpal.

Film 24 Left distal radius fracture and triquetral fracture.

Film 25 Bilateral pulmonary oedema.

> Tip: Perihilar shadowing (batwings). Differential diagnoses to consider are pulmonary haemorrhage and alveolar proteinosis.

Film 26 Fracture of the distal end of the right clavicle.

Film 27 Fracture of the left distal fibula and calcaneum.

> Tip: In the calcaneal fracture, note the loss of Bohler's angle. This is assessed on the lateral ankle X-ray.

Film 28 Fracture of the right medial cuneiform.

Film 29 Left supracondylar fracture with posterior displacement and joint effusion.

Film 30 Normal chest. Fracture of the left humeral neck.

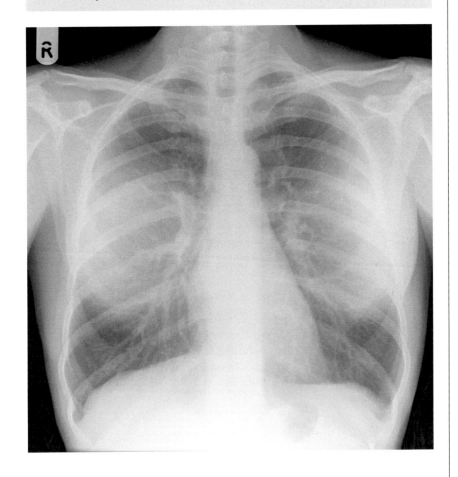

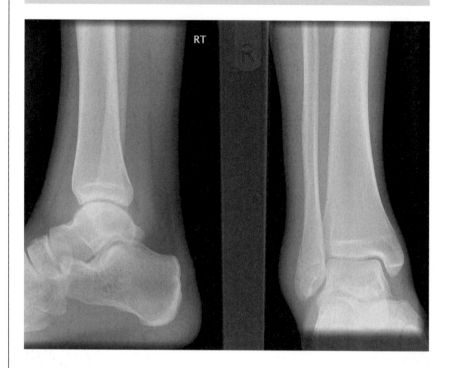

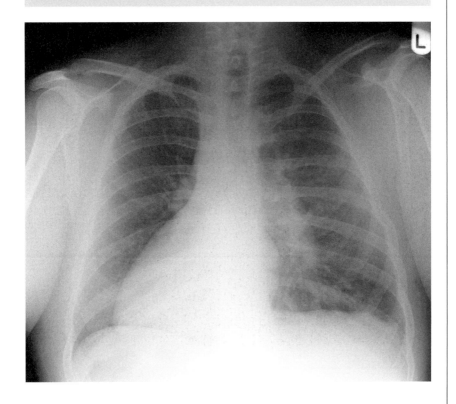

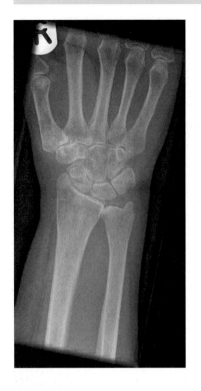
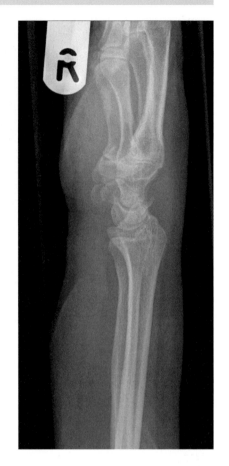

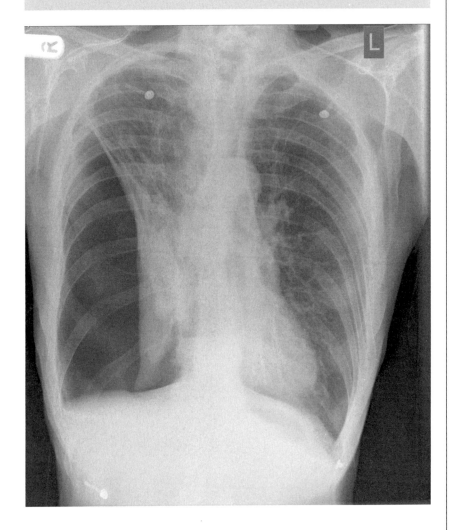

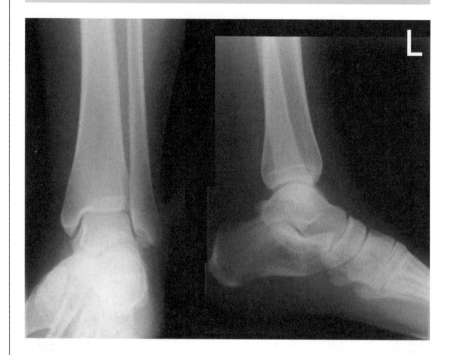

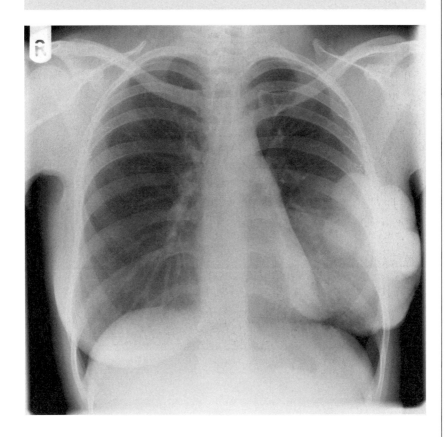

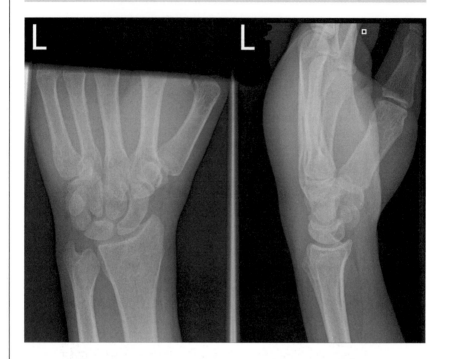

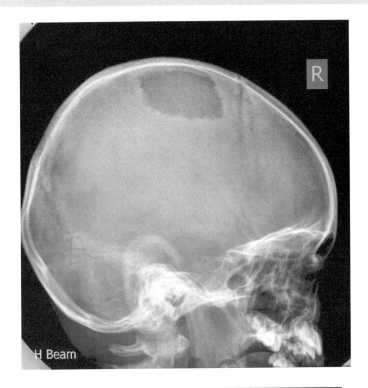

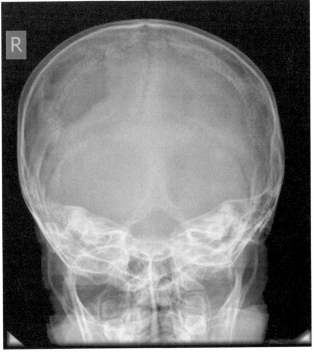

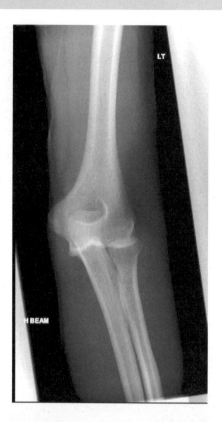

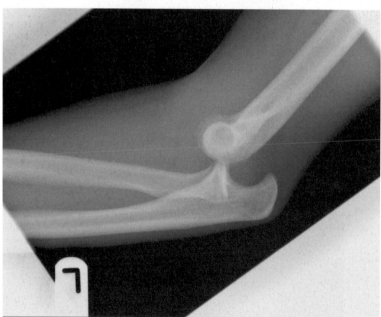

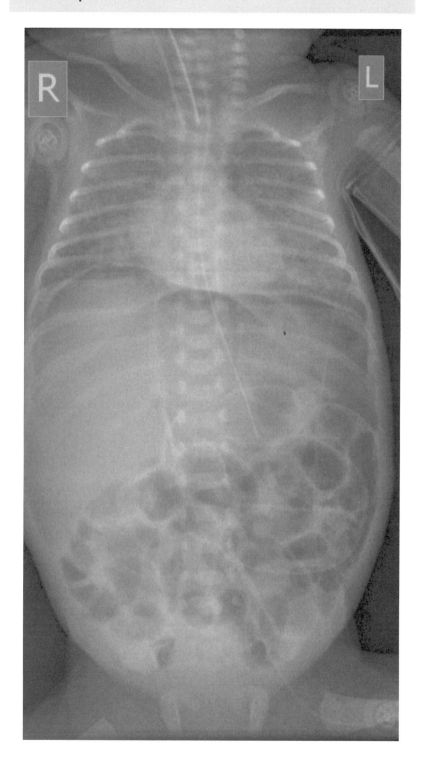

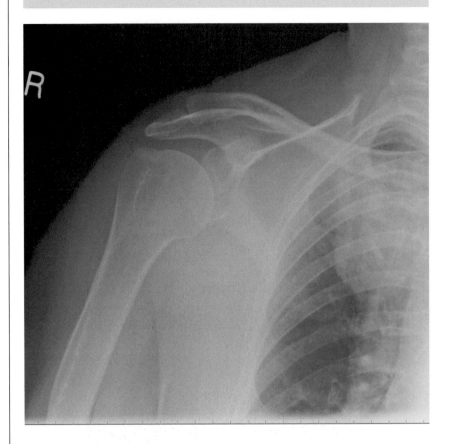

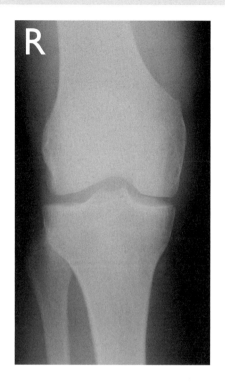

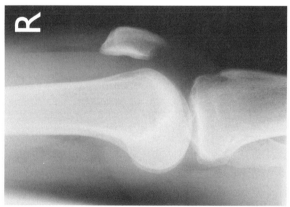

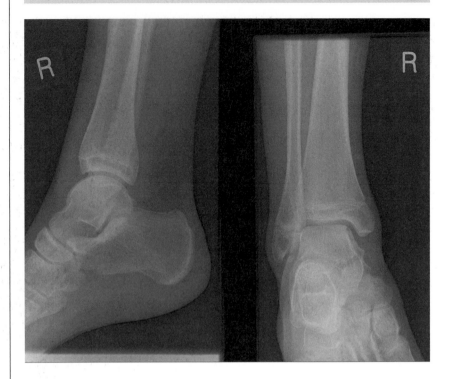

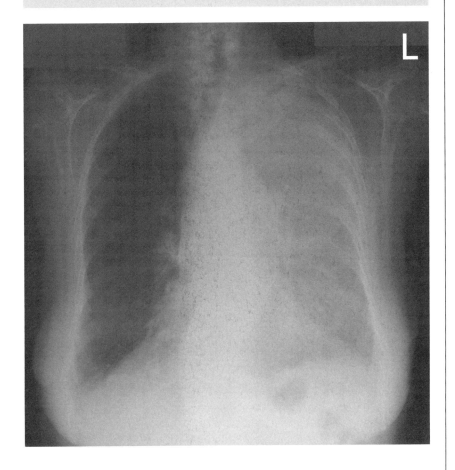

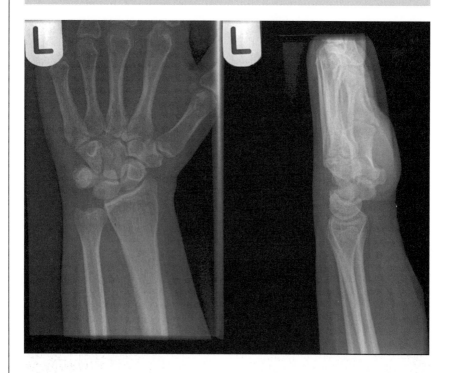

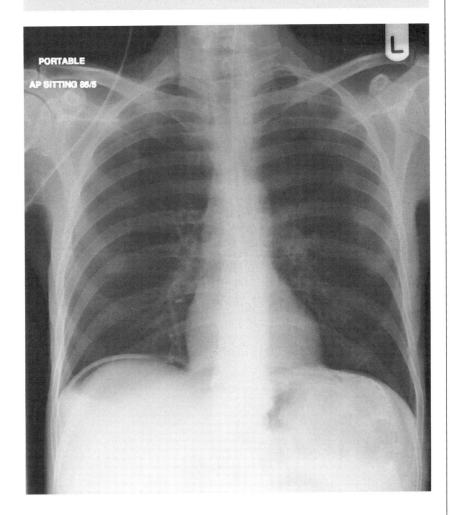

PORTABLE

AP SITTING 85/5

L

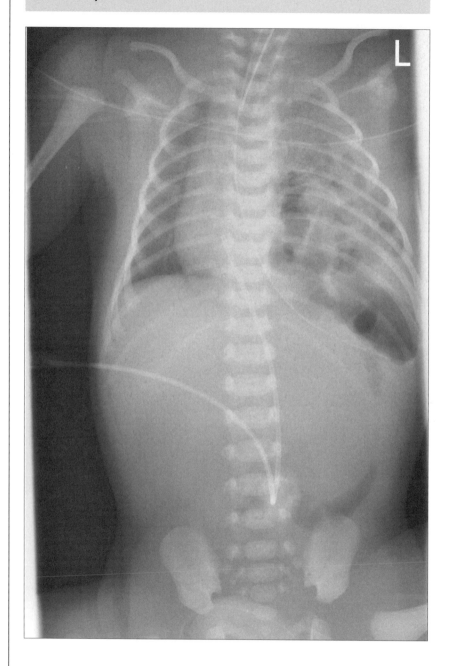

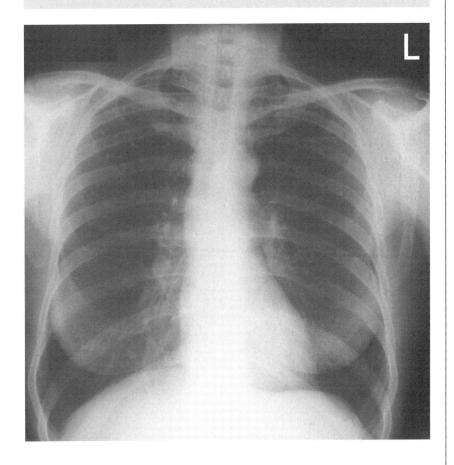

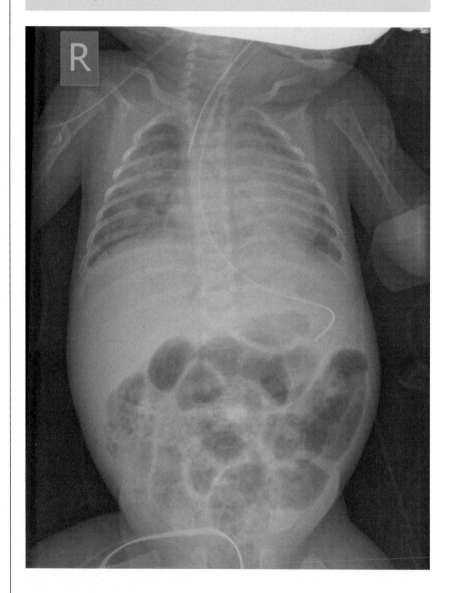

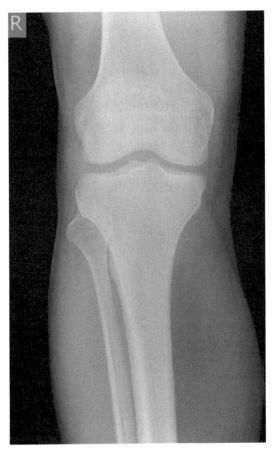

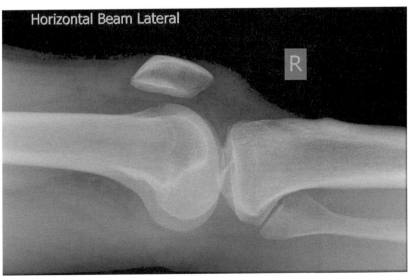

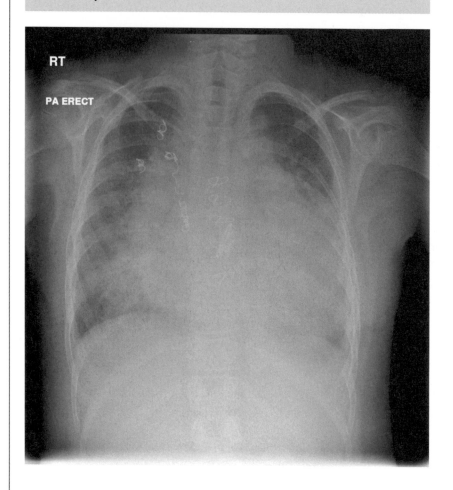

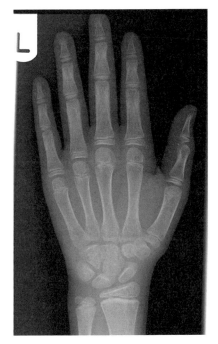
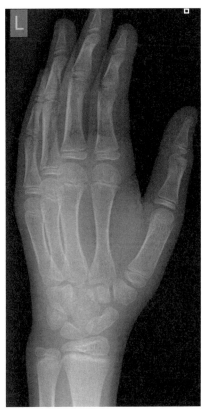

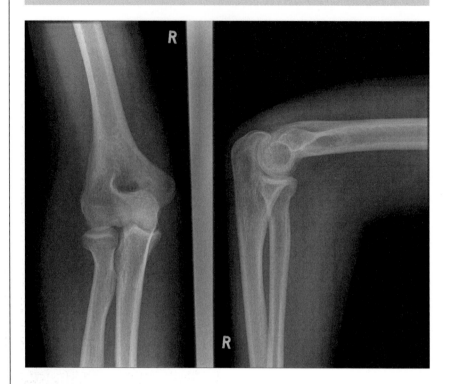

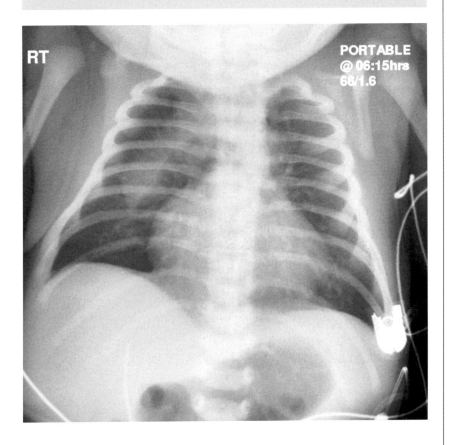

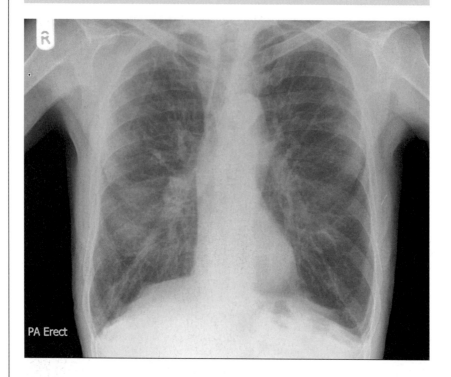

PA Erect

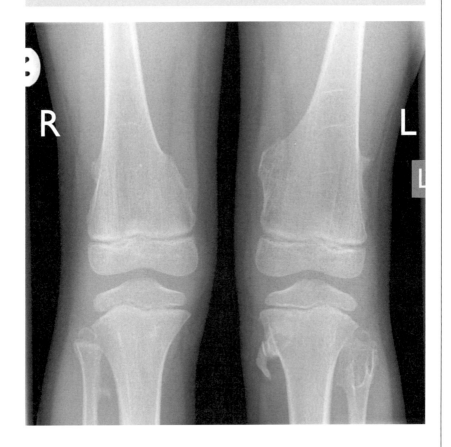

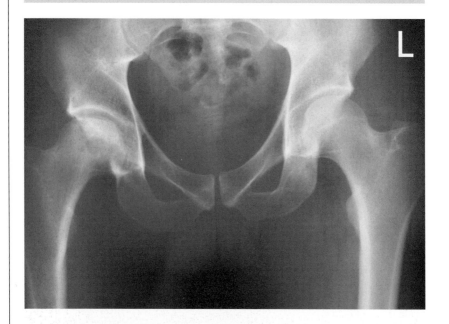

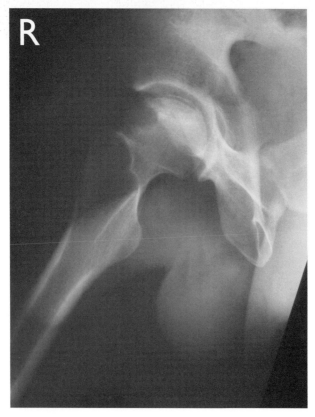

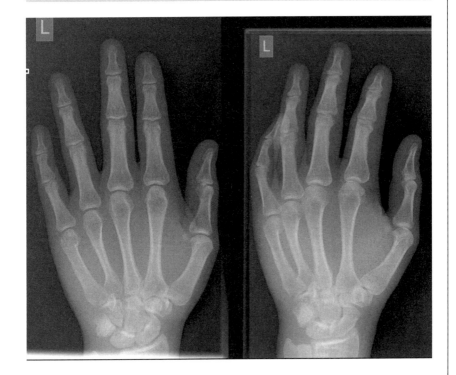

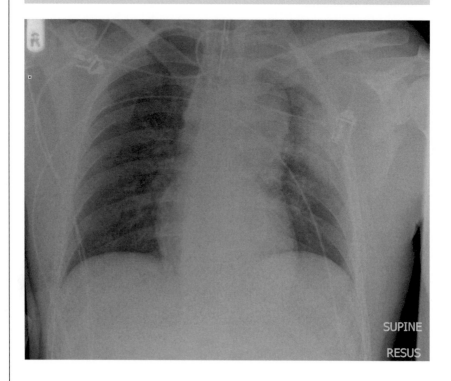

Practice Paper 5: Answers

Film 1   Normal chest.

Film 2   Fracture of distal right fibula.

Film 3   Dextrocardia.

Associations: Dextrocardia can be associated with *situs solitus*, i.e. the cardiac apex is directed rightwards and the stomach bubble is on the left. Approximately 90% of cases are associated with congenital heart disease, usually cyanotic (corrected transposition of the great arteries, ventricular septal defect and pulmonary stenosis);
or
situs inversus, i.e. the visceral organs are on the opposite side to normal (including the gastric bubble). Association with congenital heart disease is weaker.

Film 4   Right triquetral fracture.

Tip: This is best seen on the lateral view. A small avulsion is seen on the dorsum of the wrist, which is virtually diagnostic of an avulsion of the triquetrum.

Film 5   Right loculated pneumothorax.

Film 6   Normal left ankle with os subfibulare (accessory ossicle).

Film 7   Left mastectomy with left breast implant and surgical clips in left axilla.

Film 8   Left distal radius fracture.

Film 9   Eosinophilic granuloma.

Tip: This is found as a clinical subgroup of Langerhans cell histiocytosis (accounting for 60–80%). It is most commonly found in the 4–7-year age group. 50–75% are solitary lesions. The long bones, pelvis, skull and flat bones are the most common sites involved. Within the skull, there are punched-out lucent areas with little or no surrounding sclerosis.

Film 10 Dislocation of left radial head.

Film 11 Pneumoperitoneum.

Tip: On this film, the signs are *football sign* (free intraperitoneal air outlines the entire abdominal cavity), *Rigler's sign* (air on both sides of the bowel allows clear delineation of the bowel wall), *outline of falciform ligament* (a long vertical line to the right of the midline extending from the ligamentum teres to the umbilicus – the most common structure to be outlined) and *depiction of diaphragmatic muscle slips* (due to air beneath the diaphragm).

Film 12 Right apical lung mass.

Tip: This is an AP view of the shoulder, but remember to look at the rest of the film. In this film, the right lung apex is an important review area:

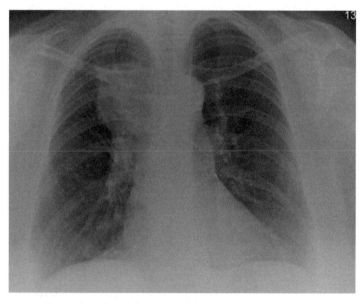

Chest X-ray showing right upper lobe mass.

Film 13 Lipohaemarthrosis of the right knee.

> Tip: This is best seen on the horizontal-beam projection. Lipohaemarthrosis is caused by a fat–fluid interface and is an indication of an intra-articular fracture.

Film 14 Osteochondritis dessicans of the medial aspect of the right talar dome.

> Tip: This is due to a subchondral fatigue fracture occurring as a result of rotational/tangential impaction forces with separation/fragmentation of the articular surface. It is most commonly located in the medial femoral condyle of the knee, the humeral head and the talus.

Film 15 Left upper lobe collapse.

> Tip: On this film, the sign is a veil-like opacification of the left hemithorax: hazy opacification of the left hilum and the cardiac border. Another sign is the Luftsichel sign, i.e. a sharply marginated crescent of hyperlucency caused by overexpansion and extension of the superior segment of the left lower lobe towards the lung apex.

Film 16 Normal left wrist.

Film 17 Free subdiaphragmatic air on the right side.

> Tip: Another cause of an abnormally situated air collection in this region is Chilaiditi's syndrome (colon interposed between liver and chest wall).

Film 18 Left congenital diaphragmatic hernia.

> Tip: 90% are left-sided and 95% are unilateral. On this film, the signs are that the hemidiaphragm is not visualized, there is a multicystic mass and there is mass effect causing mediastinal shift to the right.

Film 19 Previous chickenpox infection: calcified granulomas.

Film 20 Necrotizing enterocolitis with portal venous gas.

> Tip: On a plain film, portal venous gas extends to the periphery of the liver following the normal direction of flow, unlike biliary ductal gas, which is central in the bile ducts.

Film 21 Normal right knee.

Film 22 Congestive cardiac failure.

Film 23 Normal left hand.

Film 24 Right radial head fracture – subtle.

Film 25 Pneumomediastinum in a child.

> Tip: The sign to observe on this film is the 'thymic sail' sign, due to an elevated thymus.

Film 26 Chronic obstructive pulmonary disease.

> Tip: An indicator of hyperinflation on a plain film is a flattened diaphragm (with the highest level of the dome <1.5cm above a straight line drawn between the costophrenic angle and the vertebrophrenic junction).

Film 27 Diaphyseal aclasis of both knees.

> Tip: In this condition, we see multiple metaphyseal exostoses (bony overgrowths) pointing away from the joint.

Film 28 Avascular necrosis of the right femoral head.

> Tip: Plain-film signs are a radiolucent crescent, seen at the anterosuperior femoral head, parallel to the articular surface (an indication of subchondral collapse), flattening of the articular surface and subchondral sclerosis.

Film 29 Fracture of left 5th metacarpal neck (also known as Boxer's fracture).

Film 30 Widened mediastinum, fracture of left scapula and left upper lobe contusion. This is suggestive of major trauma, and the widened mediastinum raises suspicion of aortic injury.

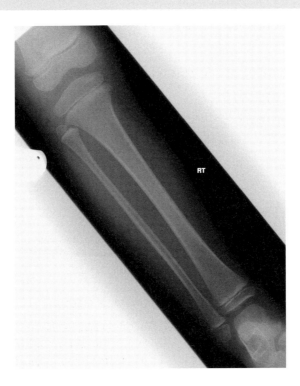

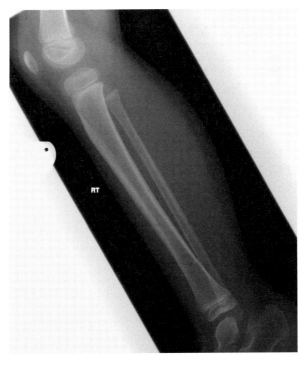

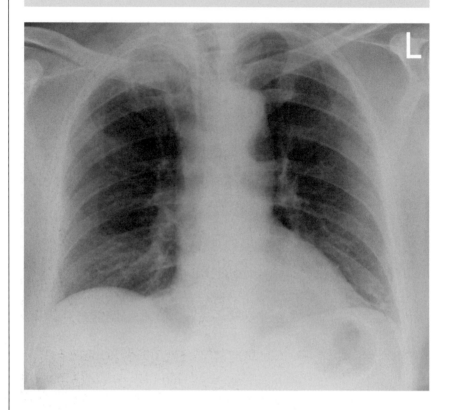

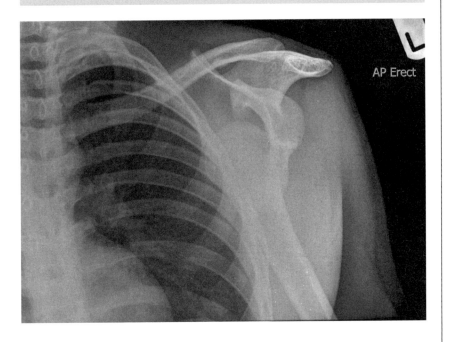

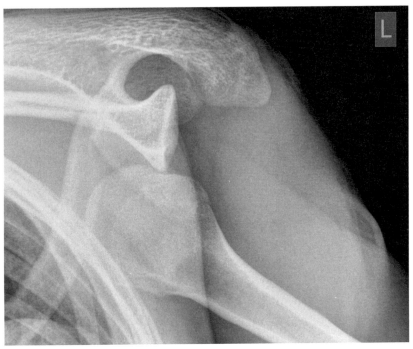

175

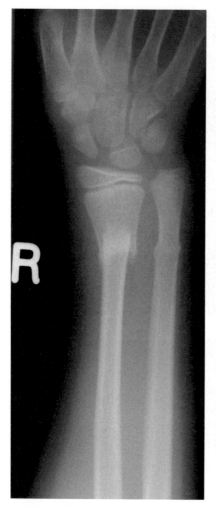 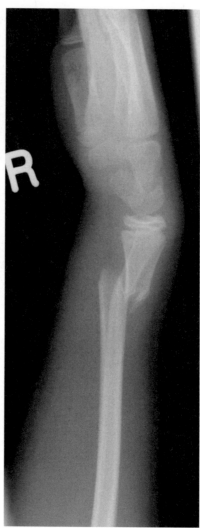

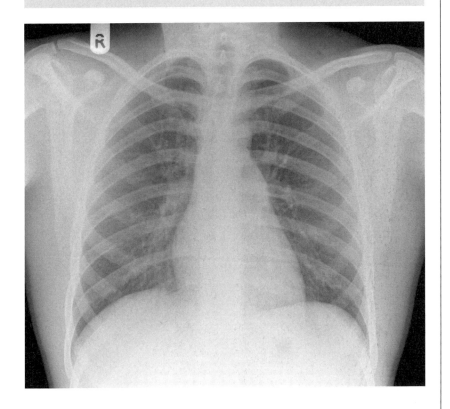

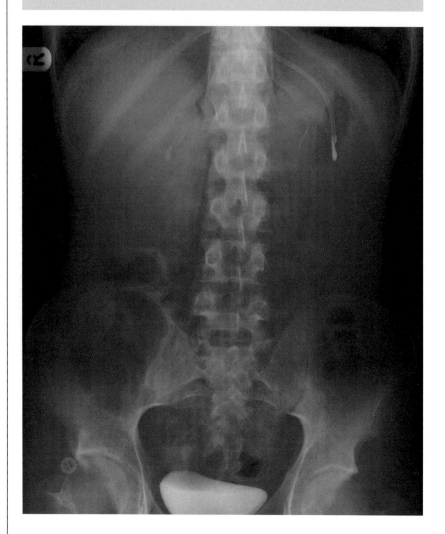

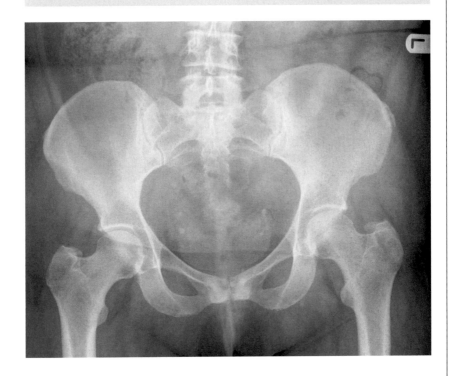

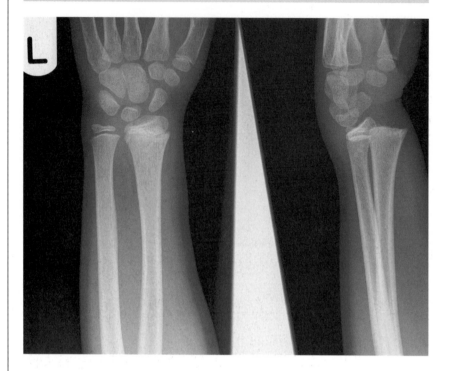

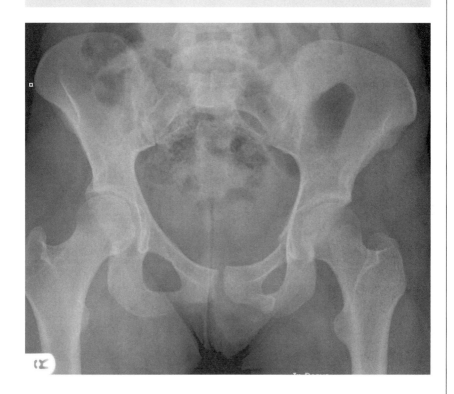

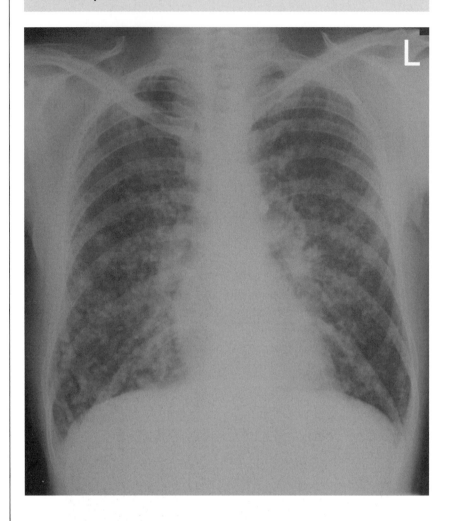

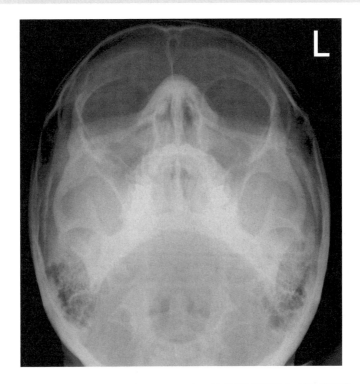

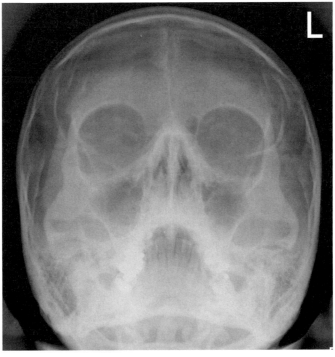

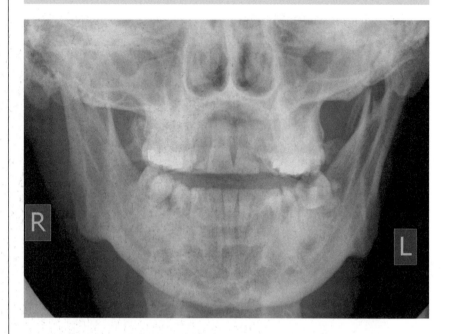

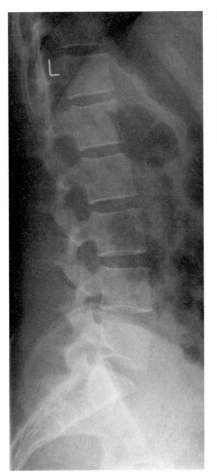
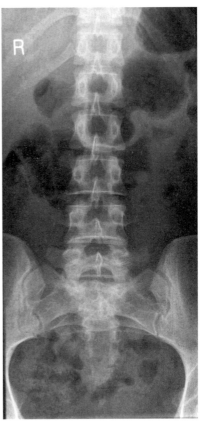

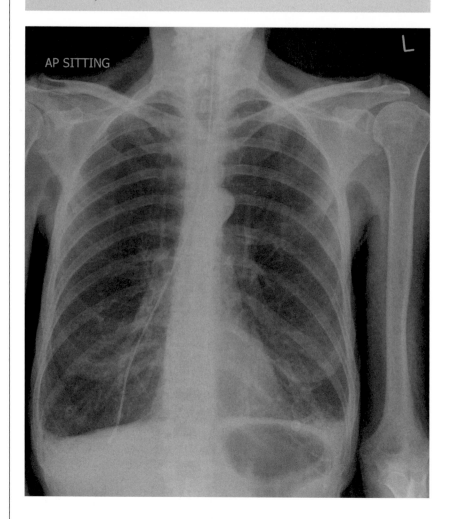

AP SITTING

L

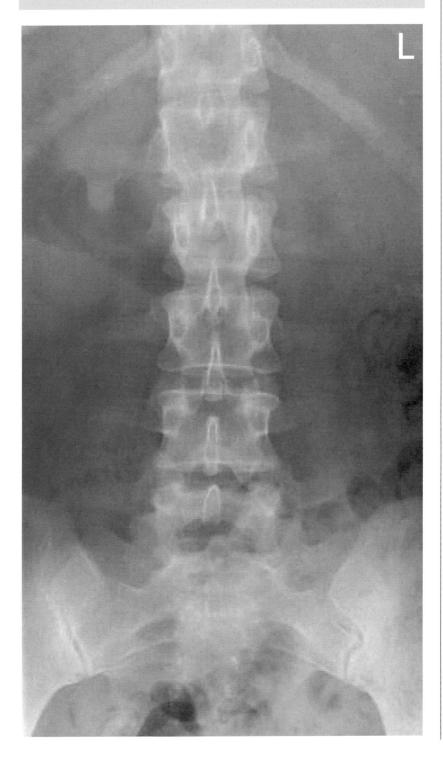

L

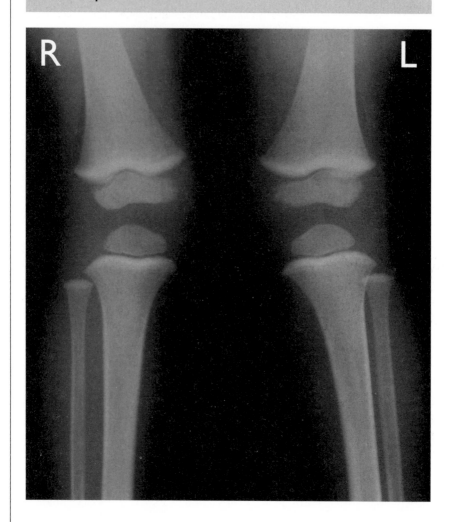

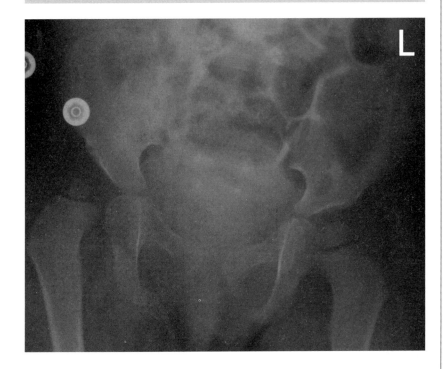

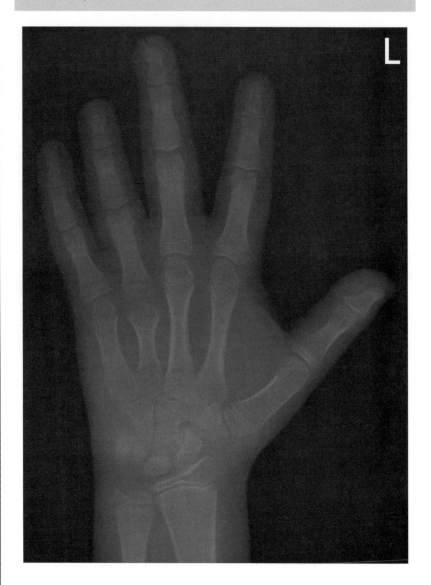

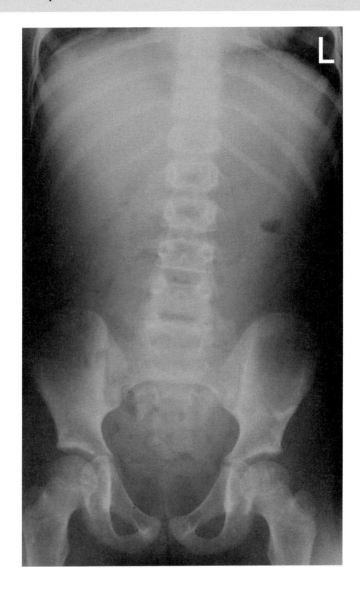

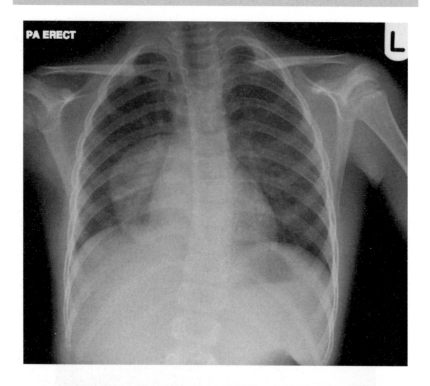

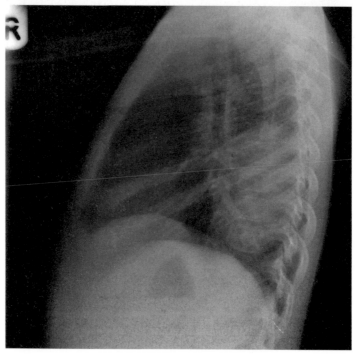

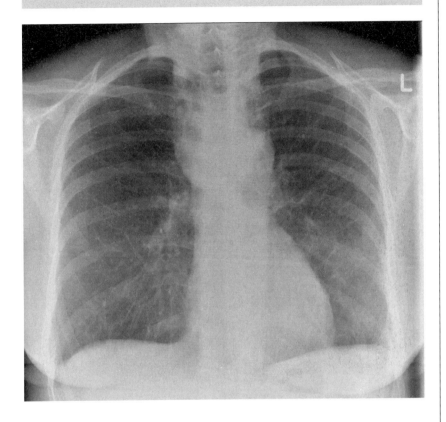

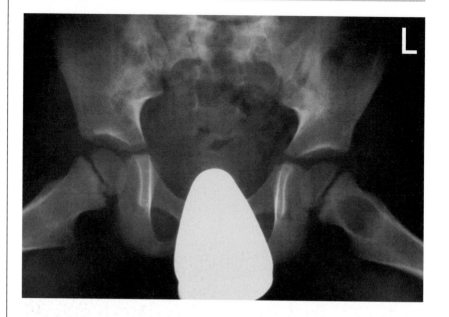

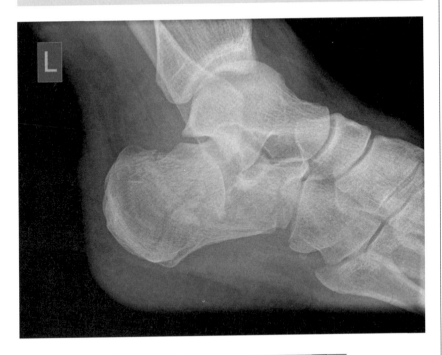

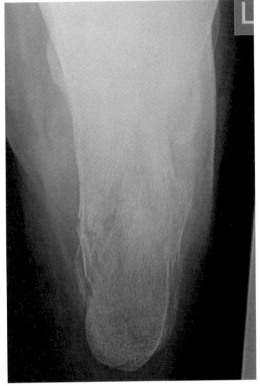

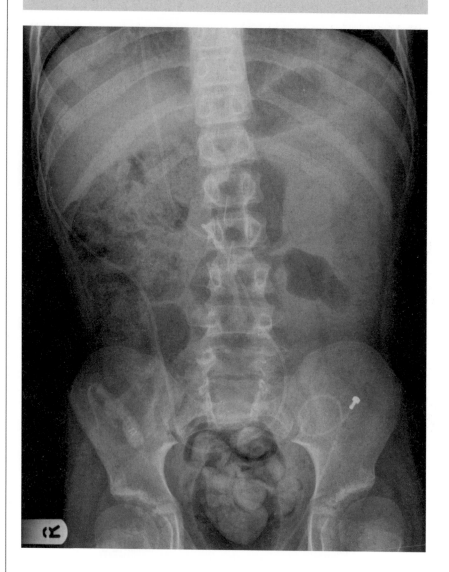

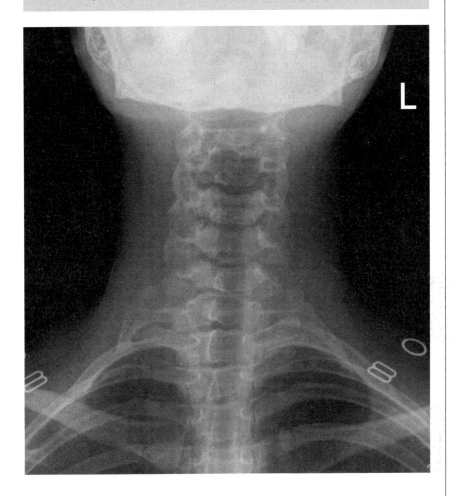

L

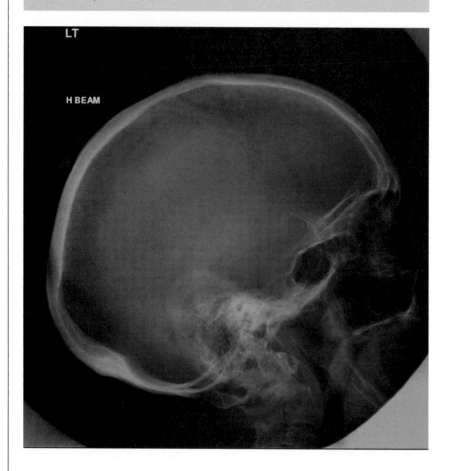

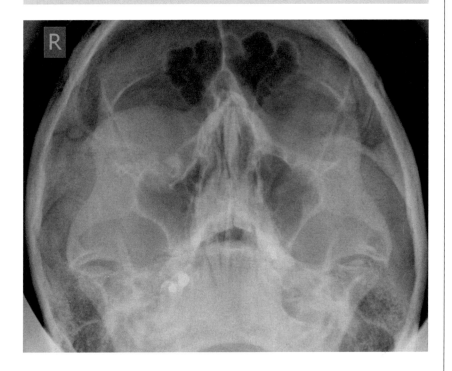

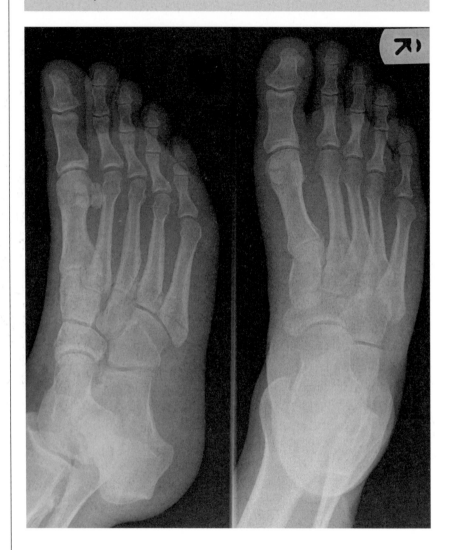

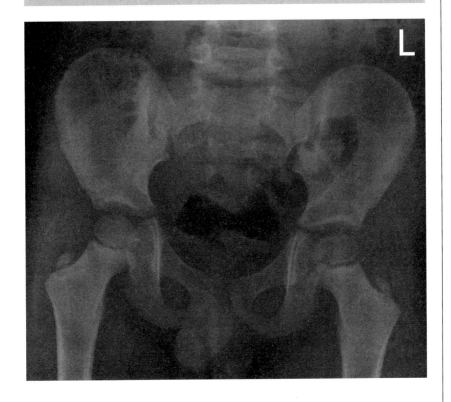

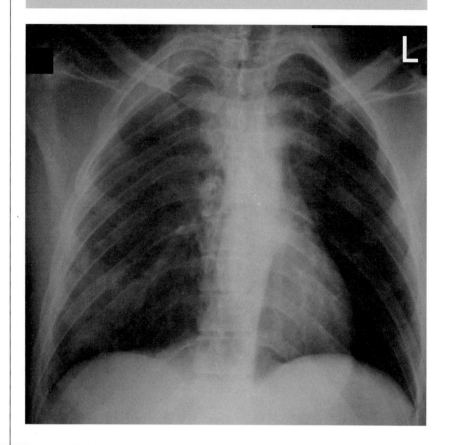

Practice Paper 6: Answers

Film 1 Salter–Harris type 1 fracture of right distal fibular epiphysis.

Tip: The fracture only involves the physis.

Film 2 Right Pancoast tumour.

Tip: There is a loss of lucency at the right apical region when compared with the left apical region.

Film 3 Anterior dislocation of left humeral head.

Film 4 Fracture of right distal radius with overlapping of fragments and fracture of distal ulna.

Film 5 Normal chest.

Film 6 Pneumoretroperitoneum.

Tip: Linear streaky lucencies are seen adjacent to the right psoas muscle.

Film 7 Osteitis symphysis pubis.

Film 8 Fracture–dislocation of the physis of the left distal radius.

Film 9 Left superior and inferior pubic rami fractures.

Film 10 Multiple widespread pulmonary nodules.

Tip: The differential diagnosis includes carcinomatosis (breast, thyroid, sarcoma, melanoma, prostate, pancreas or bronchus), lymphoma or sarcoidosis.

Film 11 Normal facial views.

Film 12 Fracture of left mandibular ramus.

Film 13 Normal lumbar spine.

Film 14 Nasogastric tube incorrectly placed down right lower lobe bronchus.

Film 15 Absent right L1 pedicle.

> Tip: Causes are metastasis, multiple myeloma, neurofibroma and congenital absence.

Film 16 Solitary dense metaphyseal band due to lead poisoning.

Film 17 Right congenital dislocation of the hip.

> Tip: The right femoral capital epiphysis is smaller. There is a dysplastic acetabulum with upward and outward displacement of the right femoral head.

Film 18 Pseudohypoparathyroidism.

> Tip: The 4th and 5th metacarpals are short.

Film 19 Osteopoikilosis.

> Tip: 1–10mm, round or oval sclerotic densities are present in the appendicular skeleton and pelvis. It is not usually seen in the ribs, skull or spine.

Film 20 Round pneumonia in the right lower lobe in a child.

> Tip: This is more common in the lower lobes and varies in size from 1 to 7cm. It respects lobar anatomy without crossing fissures. Differential diagnoses are bronchogenic cyst, neuroblastoma and pulmonary sequestration.

Film 21 Anterior mediastinal mass.

> Tip: Differential diagnoses are thymoma, lymphoma, thyroid mass and teratoma.

Film 22 Unicameral bone cyst in left proximal femur.

> Tip: This is a well-defined expansile, lucent lesion, located centrally. It occurs in the humerus or femur (60–80%). The cyst is found in the proximal metaphysis adjacent to epiphyseal cartilage. It migrates into the diaphysis with bone growth.

Film 23 Left calcaneal fracture.

Film 24 Spina bifida with ventriculo-peritoneal shunt.

Film 25 Bilateral cervical ribs.

> Tip: Note that the transverse processes for cervical ribs are directed inferolaterally, whereas those for the thoracic spine are directed superolaterally.

Film 26 Fracture of C2 seen on lateral skull.

> Tip: Remember to look at the rest of the film.

Film 27 Fracture of the right infra-orbital floor with soft tissue opacity ('teardrop' sign).

Film 28 Fracture of right base of 5th metatarsal.

Film 29 Normal paediatric pelvis.

Film 30 The CXR shows fracture–dislocation of the mid-
thoracic spine. The appearance is subtle, but note the
loss of alignment of the spinous processes in the upper
with those in the mid- and lower thoracic spine:

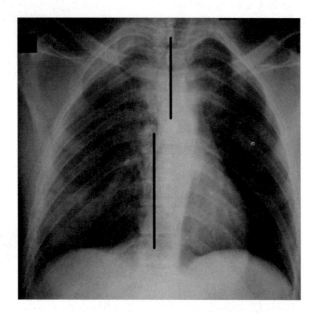

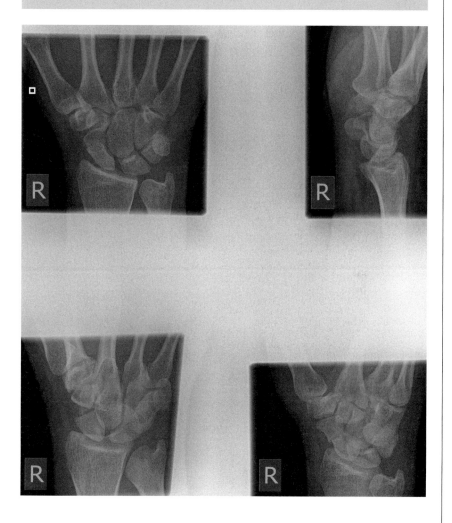

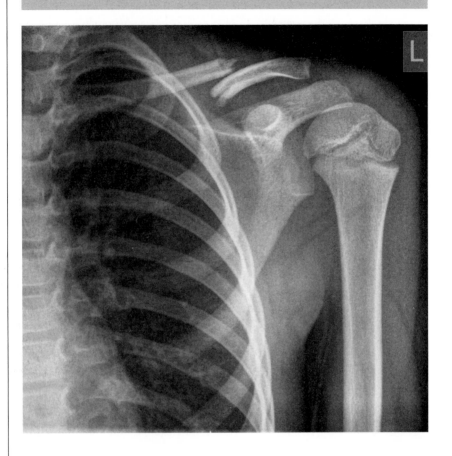

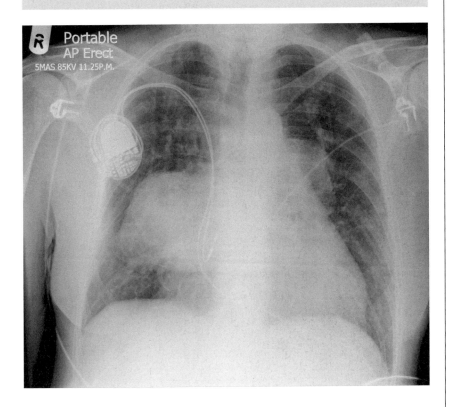

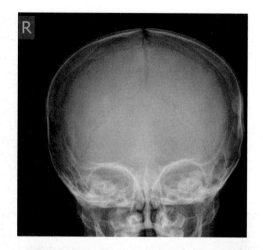

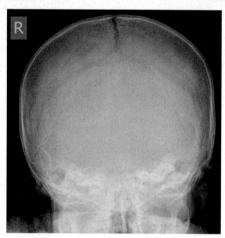

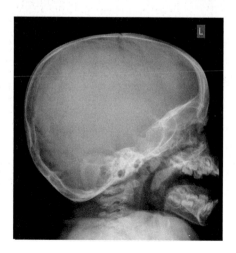

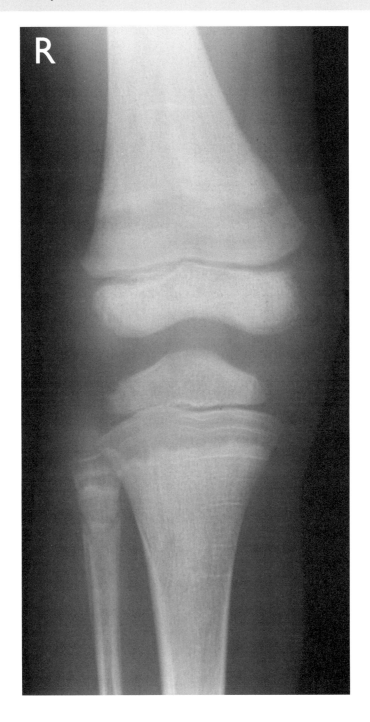

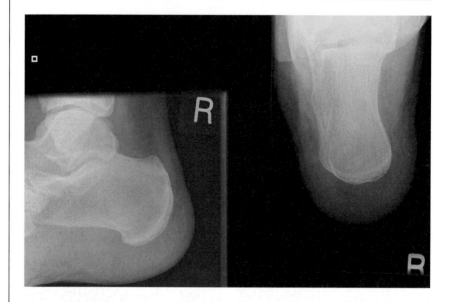

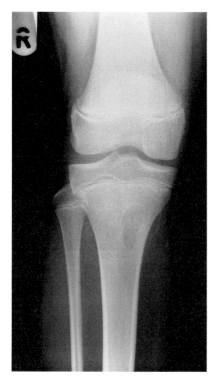 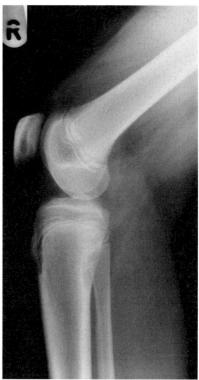

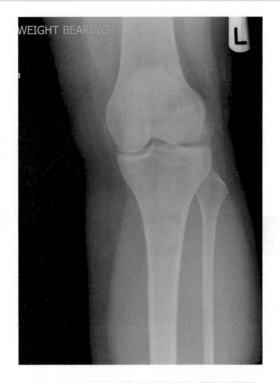

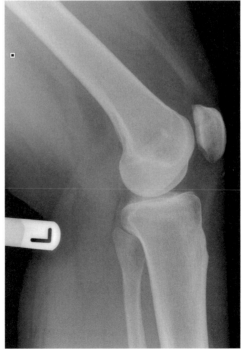

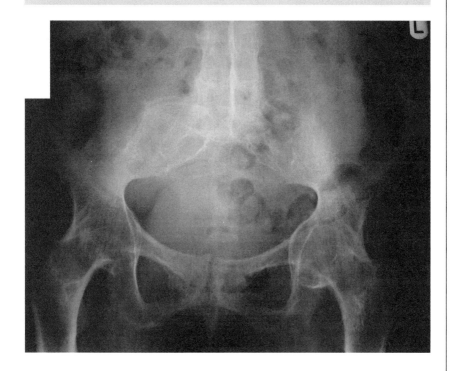

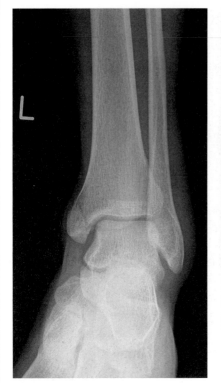
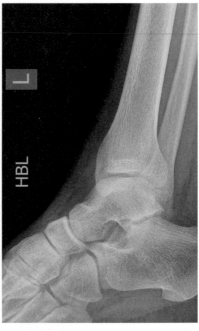

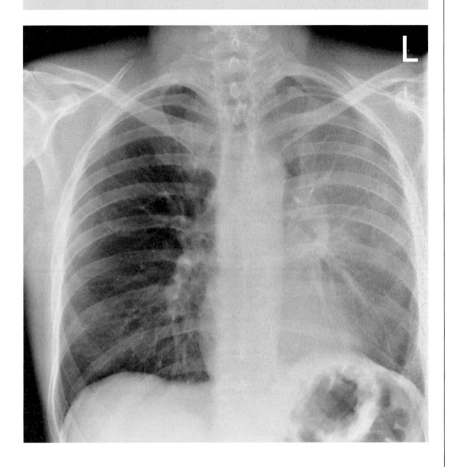

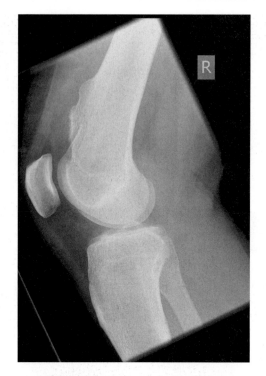

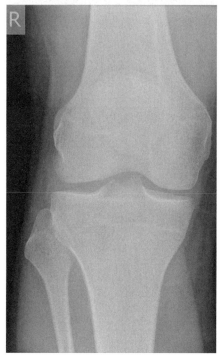

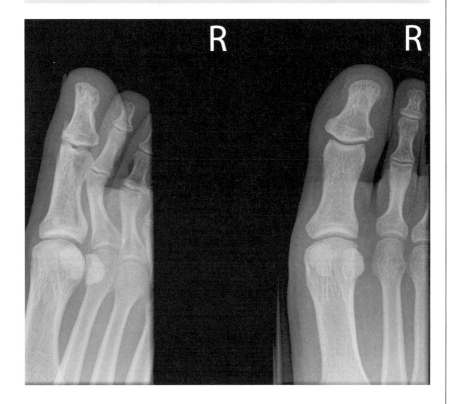

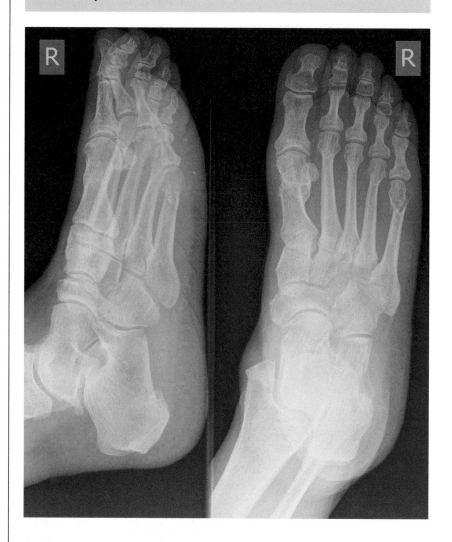

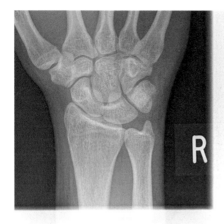
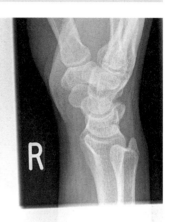
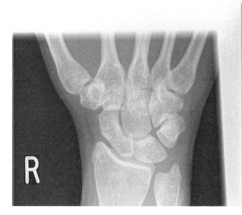
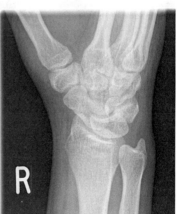

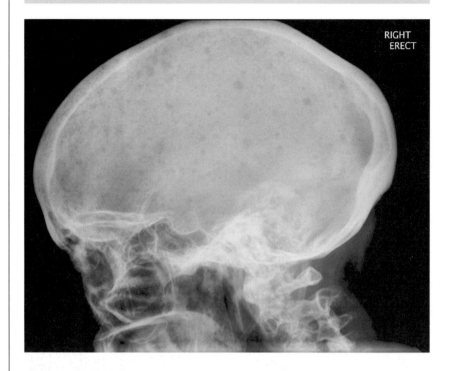

RIGHT
ERECT

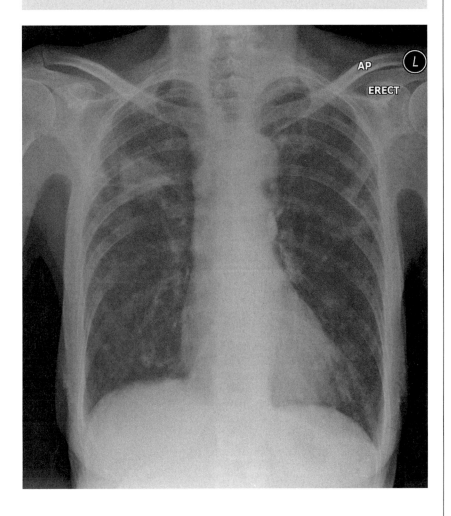

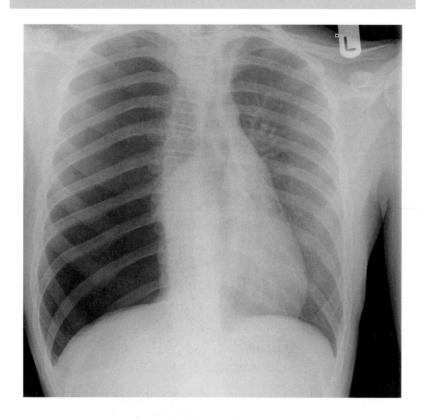

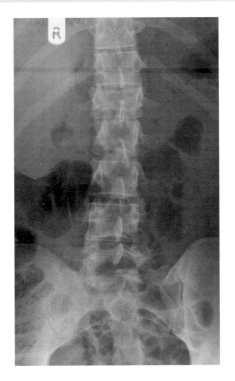

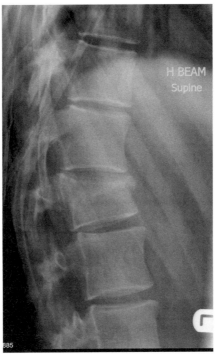

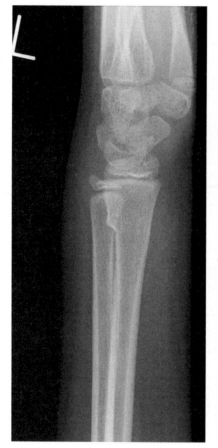
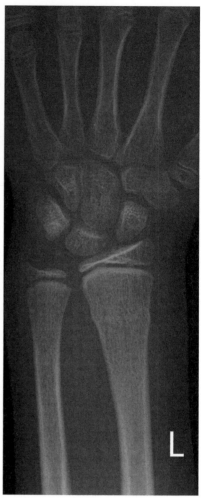

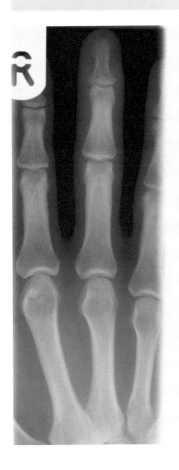
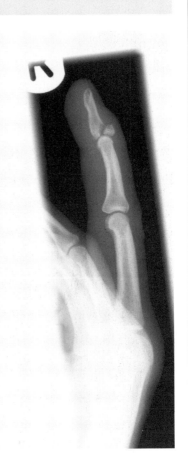

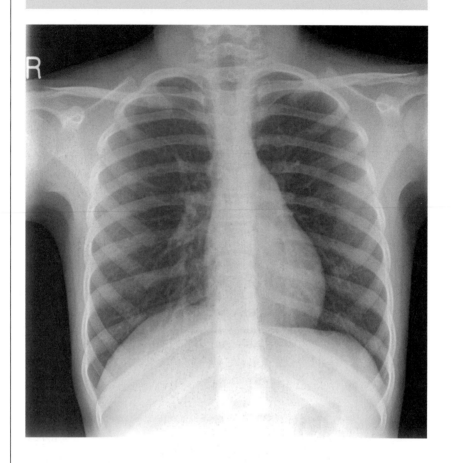

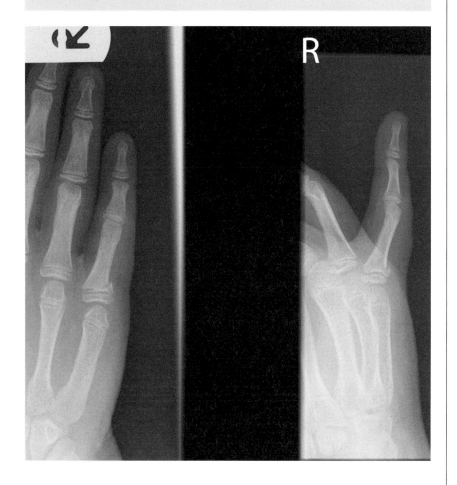

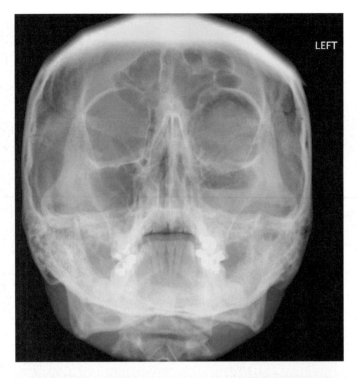

LEFT

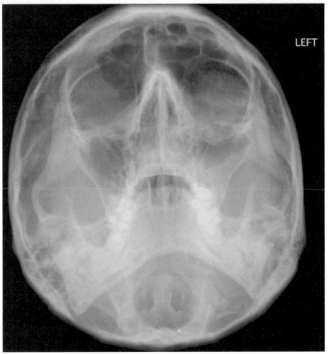

LEFT

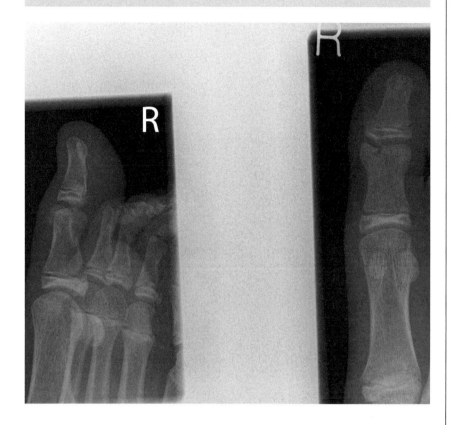

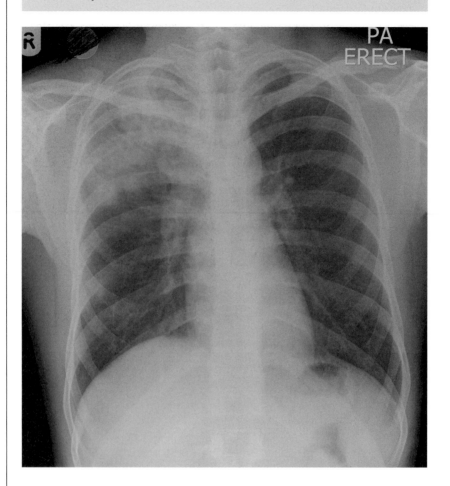

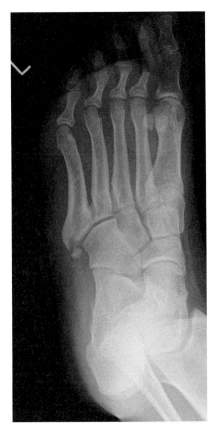
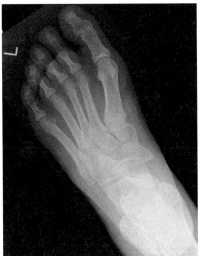

233

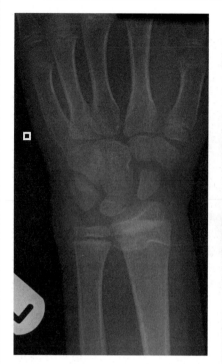
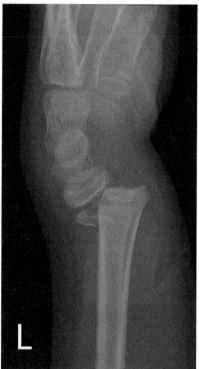

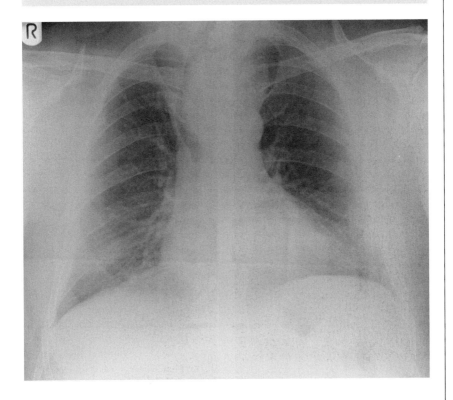

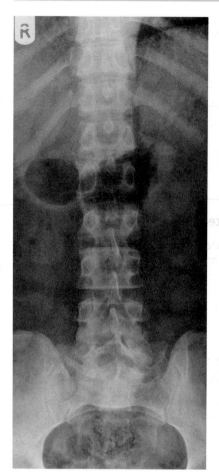
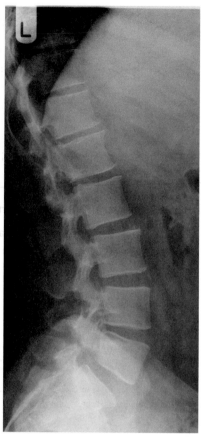

Practice Paper 7: Answers

Film 1 Fracture through waist of right scaphoid.

Tip: Fractures across the waist of the scaphoid bone jeopardize the blood supply of the proximal fragment.

Film 2 Fracture of distal third of left clavicle in a child.

Film 3 Bilateral pulmonary artery aneurysms.

Tip: Differential diagnoses are either causes of bilateral hilar enlargement or pulmonary artery enlargement.

Film 4 Normal paediatric skull.

Film 5 Lucent metaphyseal bands in right distal femur and proximal tibia and fibula.

Tip: Differential diagnoses are metaphyseal fracture, metastatic neuroblastoma and leukaemia.

Film 6 Normal right calcaneum.

Film 7 Non-ossifying fibroma of right tibial metaphysis.

Tip: This is a well-defined expansile eccentric lytic lesion with thin or scalloped sclerotic margins in the metaphysis of a long bone. It is found in the tibia in 43% of cases.

Film 8 Normal left knee.

Tip: Bipartite patella is a secondary ossification centre in the superolateral pole. It is usually asymptomatic. The male-to-female ratio is 9:1.

Film 9 Ankylosing spondylitis.

> Tip: There is a 'bamboo spine' and fusion of the sacro-iliac joints.

Film 10 Fracture of left medial malleolus.

Film 11 Left upper lobe collapse.

Film 12 Right osteochondroma of the distal femur.

> Tip: The most common sites are the distal femur, proximal tibia, proximal humerus, pelvis and scapula. It is usually metaphyseal, well defined and directed away from the bone.

Film 13 Normal right great toe.

Film 14 Fracture of neck of 5th right metatarsal.

Film 15 Normal right scaphoid.

Film 16 Multiple myeloma of the skull.

Film 17 Right upper lobe carcinoma with pulmonary metastases.

Film 18 Right tension pneumothorax.

Film 19 Wedge fracture of L1. The normal posterior concavity of the vertebral body is lost. The bone fragment is displaced into the spinal canal.

Film 20 Left radial torus fracture.

Film 21 Fracture at base of distal phalanx of right middle finger at point of insertion of extensor tendon.

Film 22 Normal CXR with bifid 4th left rib.

Film 23 Salter–Harris type 2 fracture of base of proximal phalanx of right little finger. The fracture line extends from the metaphysis into the physeal plate.

Film 24 Left infra-orbital floor fracture with fluid level (haemorrhage) in left maxillary sinus.

Film 25 Fracture of medial aspect of distal portion of right middle phalanx.

Film 26 Right upper lobe consolidation.

Film 27 Avulsion fracture of base of 5th left metatarsal.

Tip: The peroneus brevis inserts into the base of the 5th metatarsal.

Film 28 Salter–Harris type 2 fracture of the left distal radius. The metaphyseal fragment and epiphysis are displaced in relation to the metaphysis.

Tip: Salter–Harris type 2 involves the physis and metaphysis.

Film 29 Superior mediastinal mass.

Tip: The trachea is deviated to the right due to a superior mediastinal mass. Differential diagnoses include retrosternal goitre, lymphoma and thymoma.

Film 30 Pars interarticularis defect at the level of L5 – spondylolysis.

Tip: Spondylolysis is a bony defect of the pars interarticularis. It is believed to be a chronic stress fracture and is often seen in adolescent athletes.